OTOLARYNGOLOGY AT THE ELEVENTH HOUR

OTOLARYNGOLOGY
AT THE ELEVENTH HOUR

ANUPAM MISHRA
MS, DNB, Dip Can Prev (NIH-USA)
Associate Professor
Department of ENT
CSMMU (King George's Medical College), Lucknow

S.C. MISHRA
MS, DLO
Professor
Head (retd) of ENT, KGMC Lucknow
&
Head (retd) of ENT BP Koirala
Institute of Health Sciences,
Dharan, Nepal

I.K. International Publishing House Pvt. Ltd.

NEW DELHI • BANGALORE

Published by

I.K. International Publishing House Pvt. Ltd.
S-25, Green Park Extension
Uphaar Cinema Market
New Delhi - 110 016 (India)
E-mail : ik_in@vsnl.net

ISBN: 978-81-906566-9-6

Published by Krishan Makhijani for I.K. International Publishing House Pvt. Ltd., S-25, Green Park Extension, Uphaar Cinema Market, New Delhi-110 016 and Printed by Rekha Printers Pvt. Ltd., Okhla Industrial Area, Phase II, New Delhi - 110 020.

Dedicated to

My Grandparents

Late Pandit Lal Behari Mishra & Late Smt. Shanti Devi

and

Late Dr. Kirtikar (Trivedi) & Late Smt. Prema Devi

Contents

1

How to Make the Best Use of This Book

A student needs to know the priorities as to what aspects he needs to prepare at the eleventh hour for the practical examination. It is difficult to attain complete theoretical knowledge of the subject for a less prepared student at the eleventh hour. This book covers the relevant theory pertaining to the practical examination and hence facilitates a less prepared student to organize himself readily for the relevant theoretical sections of practical examination in consultation with a standard textbook. This book is a very helpful guide for those students who wish to organize their knowledge in order to attain good marks. The matter presented herewith is a boon for those unprepared students who intend only to pass somehow. Following are the different aspects one needs to give priority (in order) while preparing for the practical ENT examination:

1. Good theoretical knowledge as required for different cases (long and short cases): This is the most important aspect of the preparation. The questions would be asked as per the relevant anatomy, etiopathology, clinical presentation, differential diagnosis, investigations and treatment. The main intent of this book is to give an outline as to what relevant questions can be asked as per the case. Again it is to be stressed that the matter presented herewith is 'sufficient' for those unprepared students who intend only to pass somehow. However a good student needs to master these answers in consultation with a standard textbook in order to attain good marks. The main bulk of this book relates to the issue of highlighting the relevant theory only and its importance cannot be overemphasized.

2. Ability to recognize the instrument and to know its salient features, indications, methodology of usage, and the specific surgical procedure in which it can be used. The basic details of the main surgical procedures (tonsillectomy, mastoidectomy, septoplasty, adenoidectomy, direct laryngoscopy, oesophagoscopy and bronchoscopy) are usually asked once the student correctly identifies the instrument. This book gives the essential features of the relevant instruments and the basic details of main surgeries as well.
3. Ability to recognize and read the X-ray plate. It is essential to know the radiological presentation of relevant pathology and its interpretation.
4. Basic knowledge of the surgical specimen especially that of malignancy larynx, polypoidal mass, malignancy maxilla, sinus tract, etc.
5. Clerical case sheet assessment is a small part of the overall examination. It is required that the student should at least completely write up 6 cases including the summary, history, examination, investigations, operative notes and follow-up.

2

Clinical Symptoms and Causes

It is very important to know the various signs and symptoms by which the patient can present. It is also desirable to know the various causes pertaining to the respective symptoms. The most important conclusion of such an assessment would be to shortlist the various differential diagnoses or to conclude a probable clinical diagnosis.

(A) SYMPTOMATOLOGY OF EAR DISEASES

The ear problem can present in the following ways:

1. Earache.
2. Itching.
3. Discharge
4. Hearing impairment.
5. Tinnitus.
6. Vertigo
7. Headache
8. Drowsiness / convulsions
9. Facial nerve paralysis
10. Abscesses in and around ear/ neck.

The later 5 symptoms are indicative of an impending intracranial complication.

The student is required to ask each and every point and to elicit there absence in the negative history. It is mandatory to start forming some image of the disease when starting with history taking and for this the causes of a particular symptom need to be remembered.

1. Earache

I. External ear - Impacted wax
- Bacterial external otitis
- Otomycosis

II. Middle ear - Acute otitis media
- Complicated CSOM

III. Traumatic injury of ear

2. Itching

- Impacted wax
- Otomycosis

3. Discharge

I. External ear - Otomycosis
- Bacterial otitis media

II. Middle ear - ASOM
- CSOM

The discharge can be either serous mucoid or mucopurulent but the mucoid element only indicates a middle ear pathology. Bloody discharge indicates acute severe infection.

4. Hearing impairment

I. External ear obstruction:- Impacted wax
- Otomycosis
- Foreign body

II. Middle ear [ME] : causes - CSOM
- Traumatic tympanic membrane Perforation
- Glue ear disease

5. Tinnitus

I. Pulsatile discharge from middle ear

II. Extension of ME disease into internal ear

6. Vertigo

Vertigo indicates extension of middle ear pathology into inner ear leading to disturbed labyrinthine function. Vertigo occurs due to malfunction of either inputs to the brain:

1. Visual
2. Vestibular
3. Proprioceptive/somatosensory inputs

7. Headache

Headache indicates the involvement of dura by a middle ear pathology.

[The pain sensitive structures in the middle ear are dura and blood vessels.]

8. Drowsiness / convulsions

Indicate intracranial complications.

9. Facial nerve involvement

Facial nerve involvement indicates the erosion of its canal by a middle ear process or a bell's palsy.

10. Abscesses in and around ear / neck

Abscess around ear [postaural zygomatic and lucs] and neck [Bezold's and Cittle's] indicate the extracranial, extratemporal complications of CSOM.

(B) SYMPTOMATOLOGY OF NOSE AND PARANASAL SINUS DISEASE

Presentation

Presentation can be by the following symptoms:

1. Nasal obstruction
2. Nasal mass
3. Nasal discharge
4. Headache
5. Nasal bleeding (epistaxis)
6. Anosmia (loss of smell)

1. Nasal obstruction

1. Foreign body [most common cause in children]
2. Nasal mass

3. DNS (deviated nasal septum)
4. Paradoxical nasal obstruction in atrophic rhinitis—very rare

2. Nasal mass

Benign: Polyps
- Antrochoanal
- Ethmoidal

Granulomatous (specific)
- Fungal
- Bacterial-scleroma
  - tubercular
  - lupus
  - leprosy
  - sarcoidosis
- Protozoal-Leischmaniasis

Non-specific granulomas
- Wegners
- Stewarts

Malignancy
- Carcinomas [squamous cell]
- inverted papilloma

3. Nasal discharge

Serous - allergic
rhinosinusitis
irritant fumes

Purulent - sinusitis
burst septal abscess
osteomyelitis

Bloody - trauma
infected lacerated nasal mass
malignancy paranasal sinus
malignancy nasopharynx

4. Headache

Headache due to blockage of sinus ostial drainage as in:
1. Infection / allergy
2. Trauma

3. Nasal mass blocking the ostia with impaired drainage leading to pressure headache (pent up secretions pressure exert sinus wall).

Note

Site of headache corresponds with the location of the respective sinus

5. Nasal Bleeding (Epistaxis)

Local causes

1. Nose picking (mostly in children)
2. Atrophic rhinitis
3. Septal spur (DNS)

Systemic causes: haemopoetic disorders

6. Anosmia (loss of smell)

1. Anosmia is often due to the inability of air eddy currents to stimulate the olfactory mucosa lying in the roof of the nose. This may be due to some mechanical obstruction in the nose itself [e.g. nasal mass DNS foreign body].
2. Anosmia is sometimes due to the degeneration of olfactory mucosa as seen in atrophic rhinitis or ageing (presbypsychic law).
3. In very rare circumstances it may be due to postreceptor defect as seen in anterior skull base [cribriform plate] fractures.

3

Malignancy: Head and Neck (General Principles)

In a practical examination it is essential to define the site of malignancy and its stage. The proper inspection and palpation of the primary site is very important. A thorough examination of neck for significant cervical lymphadenopathy (size > 1 cm) and the various distant sites (Table 3.1) form an integral part of staging assessment. The cervical lymph nodes from Level I to level V (Table 3.2) are thoroughly palpated in flexed neck position (Fig. 3.1). The staging of lymph node metastasis is almost same for different head and neck cancers (Table 3.3). The evidences of distant metastasis can be clinically detected through proper history and examination (Table 3.1).

Table 3.1.

History	Examination	Distant metastasis
1. Lump in abdomen with or without abdominal discomfort	Hepatomegaly Splenomegaly lymph nodes (aortic/para-aortic) Suprapubic lump	Liver Spleen Lymph nodes, intestines Ovaries, uterus
2. Urinary symptoms with unusual discomfort in abdomen	Prostate enlargement on per rectal examination	Prostate
3. Dyspnoea, hemoptysis	Crepts, Rhonchi, decreased air entry in lungs on auscultation	Lung
4. Heaviness/ swelling in breast	Breast lump	Breast
5. Bone pains	Bony tenderness	Bone

Note

1. Always order for ultrasonography of abdomen in case of suspicious metastasis.
2. Never forget to do a per-rectal examination in case of abdominal lump.
3. Very high degree of suspicion for a distant metastasis in abdomen is to be considered in case of left supraclavicular lymphadenopathy.
4. Plain X-ray of the relevant bone with suspicious metastasis is to be undertaken. The presence of focal radioleucency/soft tissue mass clinches the diagnosis.

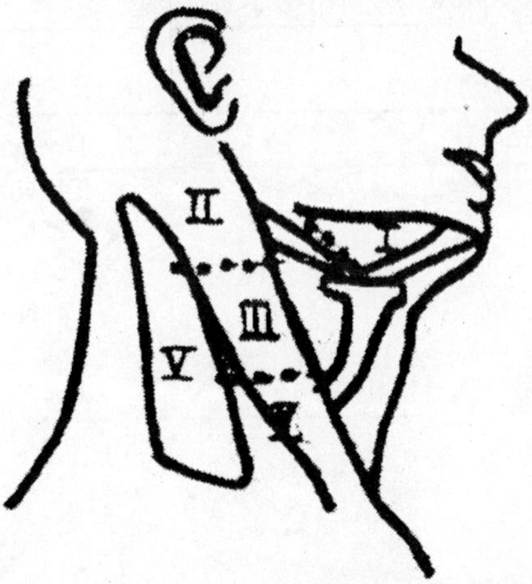

Fig. 3.1. Five levels (groups) of cervical lymphadenopathy.

Table 3.2: Levels of lymph nodes

Level	Name	Location
I(a)	Submental	in submental triangle
I(b)	Submandibular	in submandibular triangle
II	Jugulodiagastric	in the anterior triangle above the carotid bifurcation i.e. greater cornua of hyoid
III	Jugulo-omohyoid	in anterior triangle above the tendon of omohyoid
IV		anterior triangle below tendon of omohyoid
V		posterior triangle

Apart from above the other anterior cervical lymph nodes include the prelaryngeal pretracheal paratracheal [along RLN] and retropharyngeal [L.N. of Rouviere which is not palpable].

The above L.N. are examined systematically with respect to their site, size, number consistency, matting, tenderness and fixity.

Table 3.3: Staging of cervical lymph nodes

Stage	Description
N1	Single ipsilateral node upto 3 cm size
N2(a)	Ipsilateral single node more than 3 cm but less than 6 cm
N2(b)	Ipsilateral multiple nodes more than 3 cm but less than 6 cm
N2(c)	Bilateral or contralateral node
N3	Node more than 6 cm

Table 3.4: Staging of cancer

Stage	Description
I	**T1, N0, M0**
II	T2, N0, M0
III	T1,2,3, N1, M0
IV	T4, N0,1, M0
	Any T, N2,3, M0
	Any T, Any N, M1

4

Clinical Cases Pertaining to Ear

(A) CHRONIC SUPPURATIVE OTITIS MEDIA (CSOM)

Q. WHAT is your diagnosis?

A. My diagnosis is right/left sided safe / unsafe type of chronic suppurative otitis media [with rhinopharyngitis if present].

Note

1. Avoid using the association of central or marginal perforation in the diagnosis.
2. Always speak complete diagnosis i.e. if associated nasal problems or evidence of complicated CSOM-chronic discharging [e.g. pain in ear is almost always associated with unsafe variety].
3. Remember that diagnosis consists of 4 components:
   a) site of disease
   b) nature of disease
   c) pathophysiology
   d) loss of function

Chronic suppurative otitis media refers to middle ear [site] inflammation [nature and pathophysiology]. The loss of function is that of hearing which almost always occurs with otitis media and hence need not be mentioned here.

Q. Why do you say so?

A. In case of safe type CSOM you may answer "my case is having long standing copious mucoid discharge without evidence of pus or any earache. Moreover ear examination reveals a central perforation with normal middle ear mucosa and evidence of conductive deafness on tuning fork test. The fistula test is negative and mastoid tenderness is absent

In case of unsafe type of CSOM you may answere "my case is complaining of longstanding scanty offensive mucopurulent ear discharge with frequent attacks of earache which have responded to medications. The discharge has occasionally been even blood tinged. On aural examination the external auditory canal is tender to ear speculum insertion and there is purulent offensive discharge present in external auditory canal. The tympanic membrane examination has revealed a marginal perforation [mostly posteriosuperior marginal] and mastoid tenderness is present. Lastly the tuning fork test has revealed reduced ABC on that side.

Note

Ear discharge may be due to external or middle ear infection and the latter is distinguished by the mucoid discharge.

Q. Summarize your ear findings

A. *Always draw neat and labeled diagram of the otoscopic findings. Dirty and confusing diagrams only add to the candidate's incapability. The answer sheet with the diagnosis is in front of the examiner, your answer would facilitate you to get good marks.* You should answer: Sir the pinna is normal looking with no evidence of scar mark. The tragal sign and circumduction tests have ruled out the presence of external otitis. The external auditory canal is more or less within normal limits [except for posteriosuperior tenderness and congestion in case of unsafe otitis media]. The tympanic membrane reveals a central /marginal perforation occupying posteriosuperior and posteroinferior quadrants [or whatever it may be]. The edges of the perforation are smooth [or it has eroded the posterosuperior annulus tympanicus or margin in case of unsafe otitis media]. The handle of malleus is present/ retracted/ eroded. The middle ear mucosa looks healthy [or pale or congested]. The valsalva is positive [negative in unsafe CSOM] and fistula test is negative or positive. The facial nerve is intact and the tuning fork test reveals conductive deafness as the Rinnes test is negative Weber test is lateralized towards the involved ear and ABC test is normal. Lastly there are no spontaneous nystagmus. [The mixed deafness in unsafe otitis media presents with negative Rinnes test, Lateralised Weber & decreased ABC.]

Note

1. To assess the size of perforation a rough estimate can be made by comparing it with the tympanic membrane diameter which ranges between 8-9 mm. This is usually not required from undergraduate students.
2. Hence the points to be stressed during aural examination of a CSOM case it is mandatory to comment upon external otitis, complete tympanic membrane findings, mastoid tenderness, vasalva a maneuver for Eustachian tube patency, fistula test, tuning fork test, facial nerve status and spontaneous nystagmus if any.
3. Remember always to avoid the use of confusing terms like total subtotal perforation. Say only large central perforation involving the respective quadrants.

The above three questions are very essential to meet the minimal passing requirement. Further questions would assess your understanding to deal with the case.

Q. How does the character of discharge differentiate the two types of CSOM

A.

	SAFE	UNSAFE
1.	Mucoid predominantly	Purulent predominantly
2.	Usually copious	Usually scanty
3.	—	May be associated with headache and even may be blood tinged

Q. What is mucoid discharge?

A. Any discharge which is thick, viscid and be pulled into threads is known as mucoid discharge. Its presence only indicates a middle ear disease.

Q. What is the significance of the fistula test?

A. Your answer should be: The fistula test signifies a fistulous communication between middle and inner ear. It is elicited by either pressing the tragus or by seigelization in order to produce positive air pressure inside the middle ear whereby nystagmus can be seen during the procedure if there is a fistula.

Q. What is the most common site of the fistula and why?

A. The lateral semicircular canal is the most common site as this falls in the path of cholesteatoma extension to the antrum and secondly since it is the most laterally lying structure of inner ear.

Q. How do you assess eustachian tube patency and why?

A. You should answer: Eustachian tube not only provides a channel for drainage of ear secretions but also plays important role in equalizing air pressure of middle ear to that of the atmosphere. Hence its functional assessment is necessary as it plays a significant role in middle ear function. Its functioning elicitation is done mostly by vasalva's maneuver where by the increased air pressure in nasopharynx drives some air into the middle ear through the eustachian tube. The other less commonly employed methods are Toynbees' and Frenzels' maneuver.

Q. How does a fistula form?

A. Mostly due to erosion of the lateral semicircular canal by growing cholesteatoma.

Q. Is fistula test positive in every case of fistula?

A. No it is positive in only in 33.33% cases.

Q. Then what is the best way to increase the sensitivity of eliciting the fistula test

A. The best method is Electronystagmography coupled with impedance bridge.

Note

Electronystagmography records even the very small nystagmic eye movements which may not be visible by simple viewing. On the other hand impedance audiometer can produce controlled air pressure changes. Hence those minute nystagmus [not visible] elicited by creating small pressure changes [say by tragal compression] which are often missed can be detected by coupled electronystagmography and impedance bridge.

Q. How do you elicit mastoid tenderness?

A. The students usually press the mastoid process for the elicitation of tenderness which is incorrect. It should be examined in a systematic manner and then answered.
You should answer: Sir the first point to elicit tenderness is the posterosuperior deep external auditory canal by an ear speculum as it is closest to the antrum. The second place to elicit tenderness is the Macewans triangle and lastly the mastoid process and tip.

Q. What is a cholesteatoma?

A. It is the result of in-growth of epithelial sac into the middle ear with desquamation of epithelial cells into the lumen.

Note

It does not contain cholesterol.

Q. Why is cholesteatoma common with marginal perforation?

A. Since the annulus tympanicus [margin] inhibits the growth of epithelium into the middle ear, its absence (marginal perforation) results into epithelial in-growth (cholesteatoma).

Note

The margin acts as a barrier to extension of epithelium into the middle ear (Fig. 4.A-1) and when eroded facilitates the in-growth of epithelium.

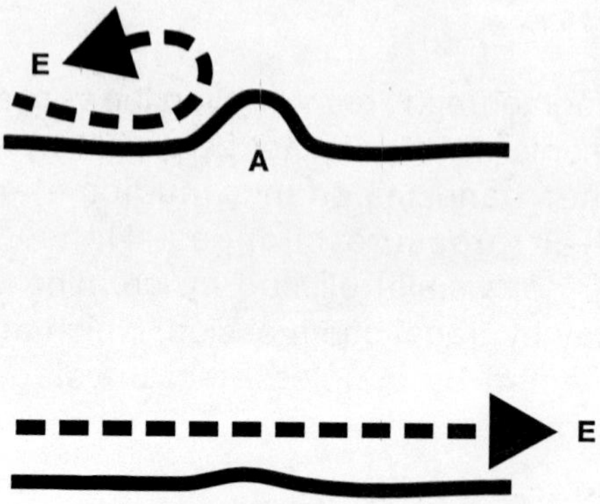

Fig. 4.A-1. (A = Annulus; E = Epithelium)

Q. How does cholesteatoma erode bone?

A. By pressure or by secreting certain chemical substances like collagenases. Recently it has been suggested that the underlying hyperemia beneath the cholesteatoma sheath is responsible for erosion.

Q. What sort of hearing impairment is seen with cholesteatoma?

A. The cholesteatoma by virtue of its erosion may cause conductive deafness if it involves only the ossicles and middle ear or sensorineural deafness if it involves internal ear by fistualization of lateral semicircular canal or by releasing certain chemicals/toxins to diffuse into membranous labyrinth. Occasionally cholesteatoma can improve the hearing by bridging the gap between the eroded ossicles [BRIDGING CHOLESTEATOMA].

Q. How does cholesteatoma form?

A. The primary cholesteatoma forms in normal ear and the theories regarding its formation are invagination theory, metaplasia theory.

Q. How will you manage the case?

A. Remember the management includes first investigation and then treatment [the students often start telling the treatment straightaway when asked about management]. The basic format is to classify investigations into routine and specific, and treatment into conservative and surgical.

Then your answer should be : First I would like to investigate my case. I would like to have apart from routine investigations such as Hb TLC, DLC, BT/CT PT/PC ESR PCV certain specific investigations as you. Amongst these I would like to do otomicroscopy to further confirm my findings. Then I would like to have the pus c/s, P. T. audiometry, and x-ray skull Townes' view. My treatment would be based on the above investigation. Firstly, I would control the discharge by conservative treatment for 10-12 days and subsequently do surgery. The conservative treatment will include regular aural cleaning with povidone iodine lotion and instillation of antibiotic steroid ear drops along with systemic decongestants and antihistaminics. After about 10-12 days when the discharge has reduced I would like to do 2 stage surgery i.e. modified radical mastiodectomy in stage one followed 6 months later by hearing reconstruction i.e tympanoplasty in second stage depending on the cochlear reserve.

Q. What will you see in audiometry?

A. I would see for the severity of hearing loss, nature of hearing loss, and most important the cochlear reserve.

Q. What is cochlear reserve?

A. It is the minimal residual functional level of cochlea which should be present in order to reconstruct middle ear hearing apparatus. It denotes that the inner ear functions are adequate enough to comply with middle ear impedance mechanism for a fruitful hearing.

Q. What will you find on radiographic examination?

A. I would like to look for mastoid haziness, cholesteatoma, and coalescent mastoiditis.

Q. Where would you look for mastoid haziness?

A. By comparing the mastoid process of both the sides and appreciating its radio-opacity.

Q. What is the radiological picture of cholesteatoma?

A. A radioleucent well circumscribed oval shadow with sclerotic radio-opaque margins.

Q. What is the radiological picture of coalescent mastoiditis?

A. A radioleuscent well circumscribed shadow without radio-opaque margins.

Q. What should be radiological picture in case of malignancy of ear?

A. Irregular bony destruction associated with haziness and loss of normal landmarks.

Q. What are the various views opted in radiological evaluation of CSOM?

A. The two most common views undertaken are Townes' and Stenvers' view although there are many other options like Laws' view, Schullers' view, Meyers' view, Owens' view

Q. What is the aim of your surgery?

A. My aims are

1. first of all to eradicate the disease in toto
2. secondly to provide a safe, dry, and self draining ear and lastly
3. to reconstruct hearing mechanisms in order to restore function.

Q. What sort of surgery would you like to do?

A. I would like to do a modified radical mastoidectomy with a canal down procedure [i.e. lowering the ridge and breaking the bridge] so as to remove all pathology and leave behind the remnants of an uninvolved ossicles for future tympanoplasty. (Table 4.A-1)

Table 4.A-1: Surgeries of ear

Operation	Description
Radical mastoidectomy	Complete exenteration of air cell system without any attempt to improve middle ear functions or hearing. The aim is to completely eradicate the disease.
Modified radical mastoidectomy	Modification of radical mastoidectomy with the aim of clearing the diseased tissue and to preserve hearing.
Cortical mastoidectomy	Clearance of mastoid air cells, antrum and additus-ad-antrum.
Myringoplasty	Reconstruction of tympanic membrane.
Tympanoplasty	Reconstruction of middle ear functions by repair of tympanic membrane and /or ossicles (ossiculoplasty) accompanied with removal of diseased and nonfunctional tissue.

Q. In case of good cochlear reserve where ossicles need to be preserved, if you are not sure of eradication of disease during surgery, then you should sacrifice the involved ossicles?

A. Yes I would certainly remove everything suspicious from the ear until I am sure that I have removed all the disease [remember that the eradication of disease is your first aim and not the hearing reconstruction].

Note

1. Some cases need one stage operation i.e mastoidectomy with tympanoplasty in one stage. If still you operate in 2 stages there is no harm, so if you are not sure where to do the one stage or two stage operation always tell the examiner that you want to do a 2 stage operation in order to be sure of disease eradication.
2. If you have done tympanoplasty without eradicating the

disease completely the tympanossicular graft would be rejected out and disease would recur.

3. Modified radical mastoidectomy is justified in every case of CSOM except where the ABC is absent signifying severe sensorineural hearing loss. In the latter situation radical mastoidectomy would be justified as there is not enough cochlear reserve for tympanoplasty.
4. Myringoplasty is justified only in case of dry perforation with preferably positive valsalva.

Q. What are the prerequisites for tympanoplasty?

A.
1. No residual disease left
2. No or minimal discharge
3. Eustachian tube patent—positive vasalva
4. Good cochlear reserve
5. No sign of external otitis

Q. What is the significance of polyp in the ear?

A. Polyp signifies the oedematous and prolapsed mucosa of the middle ear in response to infection—it indicates mucositis.

Note

1. Middle ear polyp is usually red when infected and on probing is not attached to external auditory canal.
2. Polyp usually signify mucositis but is also seen in underlying cholesteatoma.

Q. What are granulations?

A. Granulation tissue is the body response to non-resolution of infection and is composed of highly vascularized fibrous connective tissue.

Q. What is the significance of granulation

A. Granulation signifies osteitis and hence unsafe CSOM. The underlying hyperemia is responsible for bony erosion and pain if it involves the sensory nerves.

Q. How would you treat the ear granulation as such?

A. The conservative management includes antibiotic steroid ear drops or steroid ointment. Alternatively the large granulations in the external auditory canal are curetted first followed by local steroid treatment. If granulations are a part of CSOM then they are removed during mastoidectomy.

Q. How does the facial nerve get involved in the chronic ear disease and how do you see for its functions?

A. The bony facial canal can get eroded by the growing cholesteatoma and hence the nerve is likely to get involved. [For assessment of functions you should consult a textbook.]

Q. What are the complications of CSOM?

A. Complications of CSOM can be.

1. Extracranial	**2. Intracranial**
A. Intratemporal 1. Acute mastoiditis 2. Labyrinthitis 3. Petrositis (Gradenigo syndrome) 4. Facial nerve paralysis **B. Extratemporal: subperiosteal abscess** 1. Post auricular 2. Lucs 3. Bezold's 4. Citelli's	1. Extradural abscess. 2. Subdural abscess. 3. Meningitis. 4. Encephalitis. 5. Sigmoid sinus thrombosis 6. Brain abscess (temporal lobe or cerebellum. 7. Otic hydrocephalus

(B) CONGENITAL EAR DEFORMITY

The congenital ear deformity mainly anotia / microtia are not very common in examination but are occasionally kept as a short case.

Q. What is your diagnosis?

A. The answer should be complete i.e. it should clarify, the situation of pinna and external auditory canal hence you should say the diagnosis as either:

(a) Anotia / Microtia with obliteration of external auditory canal (here no opening of external auditory canal seen).

(b) Anotia / Microtia with stenosed external auditory canal (here the opening of external auditory canal is reduced).

(c) Simply saying anotia or microtia would mean that auditory canal is normal.

Q. What are the grades of Microtia?

A. There are 3 grades of Microtia:

Grade 1. deformed pinna with most of the structures identifiable

Grade 2. deformed pinna with some of structures identifiable

Grade 3. none of the structural identifiable. (i.e. ANOTIA)

Note

The grades of above degrees of microtia can be mentioned in the diagnosis as well.

Q. What are the various structures of pinna?

A. They are (helix, antihelix, tragus, antitragus & lobule).

Q. What is the etiology of microtia (or why does it occur)?

A. The development of pinna is from 6 tubercles that fuse to from the pinna if the fusion is incomplete or improper then microtia results.

It is often possible to see the preauricular tags signifying incomplete fusion of these tubercles.

Q. What are the other congenital anomalies of external ear?

A. The various congenital anomalies of pinna may be related to (1) variation in shape, for example, bat ears. (2) complete or partial absence of pinna (anotia /microtia) (3) accessory single /multiple ear (4) preauricular sinus (5) congenital atresia (obliteration) of external auditory canal.

Q. How would you investigate a case of microtia with obliteration of external auditory canal?

A. We should investigate the hearing function status and subject the ear for CT/MRI scanning to see the structural deformity.

Q. How would you treat the case?

A. In unilateral pathology with the other ear being normal, no surgical management is indicated till the individual is 17 years of age (to take his / her own decision as any surgery would involve the risk of facial nerve damage). In bilateral involvement, stress is to be given to the degree of functional impairment. If the inner ear is near normal, surgery is undertaken for recanalizing the external auditory canal and reconstructing the middle ear.

The reconstruction of pinna is taken up later in the late adolescent or adult life. The use of hearing aids especially the bone conductor ones are indicated in bilateral inner ear malformation, however the air conduction aids may be used postoperatively in order to enhance the hearing functions.

(C) PREAURICULAR SINUS

Q. What is your diagnosis?

A. My diagnosis is preauricular sinus (remember to add prefix 'infected' if so).

Q. How does it arise (what is the etiology)?

A. It is the remnant of lst branchial cleft and denotes incomplete fusion.

Q. How will you manage the case?

A. Firstly, I would like to investigate the case in terms of culture and sensitivity (if infected only) and to undertake a sinogram to know the extent of sinus after controlling the infection.
After controlling infection we will excise the sinus tract,

Note

If preauricular sinus is not infected and asymptomatic then it can be left as such, till it becomes problematic. However, it should be preferably excised if the patient is willing to undergo surgery.

(D) DEVIATED NASAL SEPTUM (DNS)

DNS produces nasal obstruction or epistaxis in some cases and predispose the individual to recurrent attacks of allergic rhinitis with or without sinusitis.

Q. What is your diagnosis?

A. My diagnosis is 'c' or 's' shaped deviated nasal septum on left (or right) side with raw area of the deviated part (occasionally present in cases of epistaxis) of septum, with inferior turbinate hypertrophy, associated with rhinitis.

Q. What is the etiology of DNS (how does it occur)?

A. The most common etiology implicated in DNS is external trauma. This leads more commonly to fracture of septal cartilage and less of commonly to dislocation of septal cartilage from maxillary crest. The fractured segments overlap one another and following healing present as central thickening with irregular deviation. The cartilaginous dislocation on the other hand projects to opposite side.

Q. What are the types of DNS?

A. The deviation may be localized (septal spur) or generalized ('c' shaped or 's' shaped bilaterally).

Note

The types of deviation should preferably be mentioned in diagnosis.

Q. Why and how does DNS lead to headache?

A. The headache is due to blockage of sinus ostial opening leading to sinus headache. Initially the patient complains of persistent unilateral nasal obstruction and occasional headache. Later on nasal blockade becomes bilateral due to compensatory hypertrophy of inferior turbinate of the opposite side. This nasal blockade results in blockade of ostial openings of maxillary and frontal sinuses leading to pent up secretions which exert pressure on to the sinus walls and thereby resulting into unilateral or bilateral headache accordingly.

Q. Is DNS always associated with external nasal deformity?

A. External nasal deformity is frequently encountered with deviation but is not always so. The deformities may be a nasal hump, tip deformity, crooked nose etc.

Q. How will you judge if the deviation is localized to cartilaginous part or the bony part of septum?

A. The deviation anterior to an imaginary line drawn from the root of nose to the nasal_spine, involve the cartilaginous part while posteriorly located deviations signify bony septal involvement.

Q. How will you investigate the case?

A. Apart from routine investigations such as Hb, TLC, DLC, ESR, PCV, BT/CT etc, I would like to have a plain X-ray of paranasal sinus specially occipitomental & occipitofrontal views. This is to see for the involvement of sinuses. A routine nasal endoscopy would also be indicated in the case where there is history of recurrent epistaxis and/or sinugenic headache.

Q. What is the anatomy of nasal septum?

A. The nasal septum is composed anteriorly by quadrangular septal cartilage, posteriorly by vomer and perpendicular plate of ethmoid and anteroinferiorly by maxillary crest.

Q. How will you treat this case?

A. The answer should be along the following algorithm (Table 4.D-1 & 4.D-2).

Table 4.D-1:

ASYMPTOMATIC	**No treatment**
SYMPTOMATIC	Age < 17 years:
• Nasal obstruction	Conservative treatment to be preferred; avoid surgical treatment
• Recurrent sinus headache	Age > 17 years: surgical treatment to be given if no response with conservative
• Epistaxis	treatment.

Table 4.D-2: TREATMENT MODALITIES

CONSERVATIVE	**SURGICAL**
• Topical decongestants	• Septoplasty
• Topical lubricants (for epistaxis)	• SMR (submucous resection)

Q. What are the complications encountered following acute trauma to nasal septum?

A. The most common acute problems are epistaxis, septal hematoma and cartilaginous dislocation.

Q. What is the site of the bleeding in epistaxis?

A. The main site of bleeding is the 'Little's area' anteriorly and Kiesselbach's plexus posteriorly (for arterial anastomosis detail refer to textbook).

(E) NASAL POLYP

Q. What is a polyp?

A. Polyp is edematous and hypertrophied mucosa and submucosal tissue presenting as a mass lesion.

Q. How many types of polyps do you know?

A. Clinically there are 2 types of polyps: if the hypertrophied oedematous muscosa of maxillary sinus prolapses in the nasal cavity to present like a mass, it is called as antrochoanal (presenting in posterior choana) or antronasal (presenting anteriorly towards vestibule). On the other hand the mucosa of ethmoidal sinus can present as a polyp as well. However if a polyp does not present externally in the nose but is visualized on X-ray inside the maxillary sinus, it is called antral polyp. Alternatively polypoidal changes can often be appreciated on the mucosa of turbinates as well. Clinically the ethmoidal polyp and antrochoanal polyp present in the lateral wall of nose through the middle meatus region.

Q. Why do polyps occur / arise?

A. The basic cause of polyp is allergic inflammation. The normal respiratory mucosa (ciliated columnar epithelium) is challenged by allergens and it is due to this atmospheric irritation that the former epithelium undergoes metaplasia to squamous epithelium. The submucosa becomes infiltrated with eosinophils and chronic inflammatory cells and subsequently balloons out due to collection of serous fluid.

Q. Why do you say it is a polyp?

A. This is a polyp because:

(a) it is pale white in colour
(b) there is no history of bleeding
(c) there is a history of recurrent allergy as evidenced by sneezing and watery rhinorrhoea
(d) the mass is soft in consistency
(e) it does not bleed on palpation
(g) on probing the probe can be negotiated along the superior, inferior and medial surfaces only, suggesting its attachment on to the lateral nasal wall (these are characteristic features of antrochoanal / antronasal polyp) or the probe can be negotiated along the floor, lateral and medial surfaces of polyp suggesting its attachment superiorly (this is characteristic of ethmoidal polyp).
(h) This is a history of more or less constant headache suggesting the associated sinusitis.

Q. Can a polyp present as reddish or pinkish mass?

A. In case of associated infection or constant superficial irritation (trauma) the presenting portion of the polyp can have a reddish tinge or show prominent vessels. In some cases it can present with slight bleeding as well.

Q. What are the situations where we should suspect malignancy?

A. 1. A deeper malignancy often presents superficially as a polyp. History of duration of illness, associated epistaxis and other symptomatology suspicious of malignancy is very important in such cases.

2. If the polypoidal mass presents as a reddish and friable tissue with irregular surface, a biopsy to rule out malignancy is indicated.
3. If there is external facial deformity and history of diplopia / loss of vision and epistaxis, a malignancy of paranasal sinus should be strongly suspected.
4. Polyp present in elderly (especially > 45 yr.)

Note

By virtue of following characteristics a clinical differentiation of antrochoanal /antronasal and ethmoidal polyp can be made:

Antrochoanal	Antronasal	Ethmoidal
1. smooth surface single	smooth surface single	multiple in 'bunches grapes'
2. usually unilateral	usually bilateral	usually unilateral
3. presenting posteriorly in choana	presenting anteriorly in vestibule	presenting anteriorly
4. attachment from its lateral side	attach from its lateral side	attached from its superior side
5. arise from maxillary sinus	arise from maxillary sinus	arise from ethmoidal sinus
6. seen more clearly by posterior rhinoscopy	seen more clearly by anterior rhinoscopy	seen more clearly by anterior rhinoscopy

Q. How will you investigate the case?

A. The routine blood hematology should stress upon differential eosinophil count (in DLC) and a routine X-ray of paranasal sinus (occipitomental & occipitofrontal sinus) should be undertaken to visualize :

(a) the status of nasal cavity
(b) the status of paranasal sinuses
(c) bony expansion / erosion suggestive of malignancy if any.

Alternatively a CT scan can be carried out in large mass or where there is a high degree of suspicion for malignancy.

Q. How will you treat the case?

A. The treatment of choice for (large) polyp is surgical:

(a) antrochoanal polyps are treated by transnasal avulsion of polypi.
(b) in adults with recurrent antrochoanal polyp the operation of choice is Caldwell Luc's operation accompanied by inferior meatus antrostomy.
(c) for recurrent antrochoanal polyps in children the treatment of choice is repeated avulsion of polyp. Caldwell Luc's operation is contraindicated as it may hamper the growth of maxilla, presenting later on as facial deformity.
(d) ethmoidal polyp are best dealt by intranasal ethmoidectomy whereby the polypoidal mucosa along with the involved ethmoidal cells and their mucosal lining is removed.
(e) in recurrent ethmoidal polypi where repeated intranasal ethmoidectomy fails, extranasal ethmoidectomy is indicated for complete exenteration of ethmoidal air cells.
(f) if allergy with infection is severe enough to result in both ethmoidal polypi and antral changes (esp. in adults), a transantral ethmoidectomy is indicated whereby ethmoid air cells are approached by Caldwell Luc's approach.

Note

Never perform probing in case with history of profuse epistaxis.

Q. What measures should be taken to prevent recurrence?

A. Since early polypoidal changes are known to regress with the control of allergy by antihistaminics and topical steroids, measures should be instituted postoperatively to reduce the chances of early recurrence.

Note

1. Recurrence of the polyp is a feature of disease and not a complication of operation or treatment.
2. Polyps are commonly seen in triad with allergy, asthma and aspirin sensitivity, hence appropriate management of asthma with avoiding aspirin intake should always be instituted where necessary.

(F) MALIGNANCY MAXILLARY SINUS

Table 4.F-1: Clinical features of spread of malignancy maxilla

1. Medial spread	(a)	extends into the nasal cavity: nasal obstruction nasal discharge (often blood mixed) nasal bleeding.
	(b)	extends into ethmoid sinus.
2. Anterolateral		causes fullness of cheek (malar area) with invasion of facial skin at later stages. Skin invasion carries a bad prognosis.
3. Inferior		leads to bulge of hard palate and later distortion of alveolus leading to lossening of teeth and dental pain. The expansion of alveolus along with obliteration of gingivobuccal sulcus results in ill fitting dentures and further extension of tumor results in ulceration fungation .
4. Posterior	(a)	the tumor extends into the sphenopalatine fossa to involve the pterygoid plates and infratemporal fossa resulting in different grades of trismus.
	(b)	not uncommonly advanced malignancy is seen to involve sphenoid sinus , nasopharynx and thereby can present with relevant cranial nerve palsies.
5. Superior spread to orbit	(a)	diplopia due to restriction in eye movements
	(b)	occular pain and
	(c)	proptosis due to mass lesion expanding inside the orbit
	(d)	excessive lacrimation due to obstruction of lacrimal apparatus by the tumor extension.

6 Nodal spread	the primary spread is to the retropharyngeal group of lymph nodes that are not detectable by routine clinical examination and hence they go undetected, the second level of nodal spread is level 1st & 2nd (submandibular and jugulodiagastric group) that are detected clinically. Hence the nodal metastasis are uncommon and if present signify advanced stage disease.

Table 4.F-2: Tumour stages of caricinoma maxilla

a. ONGRENS CLASSIFICATION: Ongrens line from medial canthus of eye extending to the angle of mandible dividing the structures into infra-structure (below the line) and suprastructures (above the line) with having a good or bad prognosis respectively.

b. AJCC (1980) CLASSIFICATION: Tumor staging by American joint committee on the cancer defines the antral carcinoma as follows:

- T1 tumor confined to antral mucosa of infrastructure with no bony destruction.
- T2 tumors confined to antral mucosa of infrastucture involvement with no bony destruction: tumor confined to the suprastructure mucosa without bone destruction or the infrastructure with destruction of the medial or inferior walls only.
- T3 more extensive tumor invading the cheek orbit, anterior ethmoid air cells or pterygoid muscles.
- T4 massive tumor with invasion of cribrifrom plate, posterior ethmoid air cells sphenoid sinus, nasopharynx, pterygoid plates or skull base.

Note

With the above relevant information (Tables 4.F-1 & 4.F-2) the examinee can sufficiently answer the question about clinical presentation, extension of the disease, staging for deciding the management of the disease.

Q. What is your diagnosis?

A. My diagnosis is malignancy maxilla.

Q. Why do you say it is malignancy?

A. Due to rapidly progressive nature of the multitude of symptoms

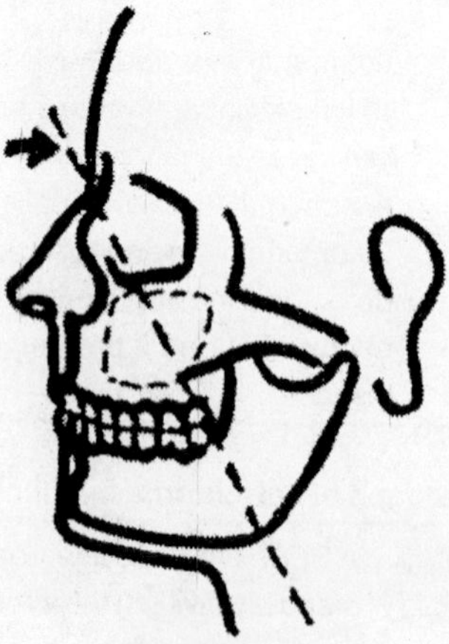

Fig. 4.F-1. Imaginary Ongren's line from medial canthus of eye to angle of mandible dividing maxillary sinus into infrastructure and suprastructure.

in a short duration and that too signifying an invasive process (nasal bleeding, proptosis diplopia, trismus, fungation / ulceration, cranial nerve involvement, it would be better to consider malignancy of maxilla unless proved otherwise.

Q. What can be the other pathology apart from malignancy?

A. The relatively benign conditions giving rise to maxillary swelling are, fibrous dysplasia, ossifying fibroma, admantinoma, inverted papilloma.

Q. What are the industrial risk factors associated with sinus malignancy?

A. Wood workers, leather workers, laborers in nickel refineries and those exposed to mustard gas manufacturing run a high risk of developing paranasal sinus malignancy.

Q. What pre-operative investigations would you do in such a case?

A. Firstly, a biopsy to confirm malignancy is to be undertaken. Open punch biopsy from a fungating / ulcerative lesion or else an endoscopic guided biopsy from an intranasal lesion is to be taken as early as possible. Secondly, CT scan imaging to estimate the disease stage is necessary for planning the treatment and predicting the prognosis.

Q. How will you treat the case?

A. The treatment of choice is surgery followed by radiotherapy?

Table 4.F-3: Treatment of operable malignancy maxilla

T2 & T3	Radical maxillectomy by Weber Ferguson approach along with obturator obliteration of the cavity followed by the curative radical radiotherapy.
	Treatment of non-operable malignancy maxilla
T4 (INOPERABLE)	Extended radical maxillectomy followed by chemoradiotherapy (palliative chemo-radiotherapy to be considered in those not willing for surgery). *In case of confusion a simple answer of chemoradiation will suffice.*

Q. What is the expected prognosis?

A. In general the overall 5 years prognosis of early cancer maxilla is around 40% while that of advanced cancer is 20%.

(G) MALIGNANCY EAR

Q. What is your diagnosis?

A. My diagnosis is malignancy of right (or left) ear.

Q. Why do you say so?

A. Since the patient is having fragile granulomatous polypoidal mass that bleeds to touch, associated with chronic foul smelling (blood tinged) discharge of rapidly progressive nature with increasing deafness and facial palsy, I would like to entertain a diagnosis of malignancy of middle ear.

Table 4.G-1: Types of middle ear malignancy and their extension

1. Tympanotubal tumor—arising from anterior part of middle ear around Eustachian tube	(a) Spread along facial plane to cavernous sinus & later on involve cranial nerves 3rd, 5th & 6th. (b) Spread along Eustachian tube is uncommon.
2. Petromastoid tumor—arises from posterior part of middle ear adjoining mastoid air cell system and the medial petrous part.	a) Spread posteriorly along the jugular fossa to involve lower 4 cranial nerves. (b) spread medially to involve petrous apex (6th cranial nerve) or facial (7th) nerve. (c) Spread anteriorly to involve carotid canal.

Q. What are the benign conditions presenting as tumefaction of ear?

A. The various benign tumors of ear are—adenoma, glomus tumor, osteoma, hemangioma, neurogenic tumor, osteoblastoma.

Q. What are the various types malignancy encountered in ear?

A. Squamous cell carcinoma is the most frequent primary malignancy seen in ear; other primary malignancies are adenocarinoma, basal cell carcinoma, sarcoma, hemangioendothelioma the malignancy of the surrounding areas such as nasopharynx and parotid can also extend into the ear, while metastases from distant primary such as prostrate uterus, breast, lung and kidney (PUBLK) are also reported to occur in ear.

Q. Why does trismus occur in malignancy of ear?

A. Trismus seen in malignancy of ear is due to the involvement of temporomandibular joint and the pterygoids.

Q. What sort of pain (earache) is encountered in malignancy of ear and why?

A. The pain in malignancy of ear is of deep boring character and is due to the invasion of dura mater.

Q. How will you manage the case?

A. Firstly, a deep biopsy to confirm malignancy is the primary aim. Secondly, a CT scan to see the extent of disease for proper treatment planning is mandatory.

Q. How will you treat the case?

A. After confirming the diagnosis and defining the extent of disease the treatment would depend as per the patient's surgical status. If the patient is not willing for surgery or surgery is contraindicated, radiotherapy with or without chemotherapy should be given. On the other hand for good surgical candidates either an extended radical mastoidectomy or a subtotal petrosectomy (depending on the extent of disease) followed by a radical radiotherapy is the treatment of choice. In case of palpable neck nodes a radical neck dissection has to be carried out.

Q. What are the criteria of incurability?

A. The disease is said to be incurable if there is an involvement of petrous apex, eustachian tube and dura mater.

Q. How will you fill up the defect caused by subtotal petrosectomy.

A. The defect is filled up preferably by pectoralis major flap .

Q. What are the structures removed in subtotal petrosectomy?

A. Subtotal petrosectomy involves block resection of involved portion of auditory canal, middle ear, mastoid process, parotid gland, base of zygoma, auricle and surrounding skin.

Q. How will you restore facial nerve functions?

A. Every possible attempt for facial with hypoglossal anastomosis is to be carried out during the primary surgery, along with lateral tarsorrhaphy for preventing corneal exposure.

(H) MALIGNANCY ORAL CAVITY

Note

Malignancy of oral cavity is a relatively common case in the practical examinations. It is necessary to know the sub sites that can be involved along with their lymphatic drainage.

Table 4.H-1: LYMPHATIC DRAINAGE OF ORAL CAVITY

Subsites	L.N groups
1. LIP	upper preauricular
	submandibular (IB)
	lower submental (IA)
	submandibular (IB)
2. buccal mucosa	submandibular (IB)
3. anterior 2/3 tongue	- tip - submental (IA)
	- lateral - submandibular (IB)
	- boarder - upper deep cervical (IIB)
	- Central part - upper deep cervical (II)
4. palate	- upper deep cervical (II)
5. alveolus	- upper deep cervical (II)
6. floor of mouth	- submandibular (I B)
	- upper deep cervical (II)

Note

Malignancy based posteriorly in tongue and floor of mouth tend to show lymphatic spread bilaterally.

Q. What are the premalignant lesions of oral cavity?

A. The common premalignant conditions seen clinically are leucoplakia (white lesion), erythoplakia (red lesion) and melanoplakia (blackish lesion)

Q. What is the most aggressive premalignant lesion.

or

Which premalignant lesion of oral cavity has the highest risk for malignant conversion.

A. Erythroplakia.

Q. What is the most common malignancy seen in oral cavity?

A. The squamous cell variety of malignancy is seen most commonly in oral cavity.

Q. What are the predisposing factors for development of malignancy?

A. The well known etiological factors with documented predisposition to development of malignancy of oral cavity are:

1. Tobacco chewing
2. Tobacco smoking
3. Alcohol intake
4. Malnutrition leading to dietary deficiencies
5. Chronic irritation of oral cavity mucosa such as sharp tooth, ill fitting dentures, chronic dental sepsis.

Note

The classical 5 'S' viz, smoking, spirit, sepsis, syphilis have been known factors in carcinogenesis.

Table 4.H-2: TUMOR STAGING OF ORAL CAVITY AND OROPHARYNX

T1	tumor < 2 cm
T2	tumor > 2 cm but < 4 cm
T3	tumor > 4 cm
T4	Tumor invades adjacent structures, such as cortical bone, tongue, skin, maxillary sinus or soft tissues of neck

The above tumor staging (Table 4.H-2) should be clubbed with nodal staging (Table 3-3 & table 3-4) to conclude final stage of disease (metastatic status should always be included if possible). Careful examination of the lesion for assessment of its extent and thorough search for cervical lymph nodes is and essential part of examination. The extent or spread of primary malignancy should be correlated with the Table in order to define the tumor stage and the nodal staging if combined with above would conclude final staging of the disease. This is important for defining treatment.

(I) MALIGNANCY LIP

Q. What is your diagnosis?

A. My diagnosis is malignancy upper (or lower) lip of stage 2 (or 3 or 4 or 1).

Q. Why do you think it is a malignancy?

A. Because this middle aged (watch for age) male (watch for sex), with an occupational history of exposure to sunlight (watch for occupation) is complaining of a chronic non-healing, painless gradually progressive lesion on lower (or upper) lip extending to surrounding structure (if present). On examination the edges are everted and base indurated. The cervical examination shows evidence of lymph node metastasis (watch for the lymphatic spread) level 1A, 2B & 3)

Q. How did you conclude the stage of disease?

A. *(Refer to tables)*

Q. How will you manage the case?

A. Apart from routine examination such as HB, TLC, DLC, BT/CT, ESR & Xray chest, I would like to firstly undertake a biopsy from the margins along with FNAC from lymph nodes (if palpable). After confirming the diagnosis of squamous cell carcinoma by histopathology, I would like to undertake wide surgical excision of the primary tumor and lymph node dissection of neck (if FNAC is positive) along with primary reconstruction of the defect. After surgical management curative radiotherapy, is to be instituted to take care of occult spread.

Table 4.I-1: Algorithm for surgical management of carcinoma lip

1 Defects of up to one-third of lip	— wedge resection of primary with end to end closure.
2 Defects of one-third to half of lip	— wide resection and reconstruction by Abbe Estlander flaps.
3 Defects of greater than half of the lip	— wide resection with reconstruction using cheek tissues or microsurgical radial artery based free flap reconstruction.

(J) MALIGANCY TONGUE (ANTERIOR 2/3RD)

Q. What is your diagnosis?

A. My diagnosis is malignancy lateral boarder tongue (or else) stage 2 (3 or 4 or 1).

Q. Why do you say it is a malignancy?

A. Since this patient is elderly (watch for age) , male (watch for sex) with a history of predisposing factors (enumerate only those which are significant in the case) and an exophytic (or otherwise) lesion that has been chronic and rapidly progressive in nature, I would like to keep a possibility of malignancy first. Moreover the appearance of the lesion, bleeding on manipulation, indurated base and presence of leukoplakic patches (or other premalignant lesion) further suggests it to be of malignant pathology. Not the least the presence of cervical lymph nodes strongly point towards malignancy (watch for malignancy spread to level 2, 1A, 1B lymph nodes).

Q. What are the various clinical presentations in which the malignancy of tongue can present?

A. ***(Remember mnemonic 'LOADS').*** For tongue cancer the patient can present "lump" in tongue or neck (secondaries). Secondly, the patient can present as "odynophagia" i.e. pain in tongue specially on deglutition; thirdly, there can be "ankyloglosia" i.e. difficulty to protrude the tongue owing to extensive spread of the tumour. Both pain and ankyloglossia lead to swallowing problems and the patient hence complains of dribbling of saliva as well as excessive salivation due to pain and alteration of voice due to ankyloglossia. Fourthly, the patient can present with "dysphagia" as well. Finally the tongue malignancy may be "silent" and be detected accidentally but this is a very uncommon presentation.

Q. Is it possible to miss an advanced malignancy of tongue despite thorough clinical inspection of oral cavity?

A. There are 2 conditions where a malignancy of tongue can be missed; firstly, if the malignancy of tongue is within the substance of tongue (intramural) but has not revealed itself on muscosal surface, it is possible to miss it on only inspection of the tongue. This is the situation where palpation of the tongue substance clinches the diagnosis. Hence examination of tongue without palpation is incomplete. Secondly, it is not uncommon to find a relatively small primary giving rise to multiple secondaries (lymph nodes) signifying advanced stage disease. Here also a thorough examination of tongue would reveal the presence of small primary.

Q. How will you manage the case?

A. Same as in malignancy lip except a CT (see the respective algorithm) imaging to be added for evaluation of extent of spread.

Table 4.J-1: Algorithm for surgical management of carcinoma tongue

T1	wide local resection
T2	< 3cm : wide local resection
	> 3 cm : wide local resection + prophylactic neck dissection + RT
T3	Hemiglossectomy + neck dissection + RT
T4	wide radical resection + neck dissection +RT

Note

Surgical treatment for positive neck node on (FNAC): radical neck dissection.

Q. What is the commonest site of malignancy in oral tongue?

A. The commonest site of malignancy in ant 2/3rd of tongue is the lateral border followed by the tip.

(K) MALIGNANCY OF PALATE

Q. What is your diagnosis?

A. My diagnosis is malignancy of palate, stage 2 (3 or 4 or 1).

Note

1. The reasons for suspecting malignancy should be framed as mentioned before in malignancy of lip and tongue.

2. The staging is to be done as per the table and should be accordingly discussed if asked.

Q. How will you manage the case?

A. Apart from routine investigation such as HB, TLC, DLC, BT/CT, ESR & X-ray chest, I would like to confirm the histopathological diagnosis by lymph nodes (if palpable). After confirming the diagnosis the primary treatment would be surgery (radiotherapy in advanced malignancy). A wide radical resection of the primary along with the underlying involved bone is to be undertaken along with neck dissection if the lymph nodes are palpable.

Table 4.K-1: Algorithm for surgical treatment palate

Small lesion	wide local resection of primary along with underlying bone followed by radiotherapy
Moderate to large	wide resection with inferior partial maxillectomy followed by radiotherapy
Very extensive lesion in a moribund patient	radiotherapy with or without palliative surgery with or without chemotherapy.

Note

Positive neck nodes should be dealt with radical neck dissection followed by radiotherapy to take care of occult metastasis.

Q. How will you close the defect of the palate that has been made surgically?

A. By means of an obturator.

(L) MALIGNANCY BUCCAL MUCOSA

1. *The diagnosis should be described as in previous categories.*
2. *The reasons for suspecting malignancy should be framed as in previous categories.*
3. *The staging is to be done as per the table and be discussed accordingly if asked.*

Q. How will you manage the case?

A. To be framed as in carcinoma lip and see algorithm for surgical treatment (Table 4.L-1).

Table 4L-1: Alogrithm for surgical treatment of carnicoma buccal mucosa.

Small mucosal lesion	Local wide excision + RT
Wide extensive / infiltrative lesion	Wide radical enbloc resection of the involved structures (including maxillectomy or mandibulectomy or glossectomy as per the case) with radical neck dissection for involved lymph nodes followed by curative radiotherapy.

Note

Positive neck nodes are treated by radical neck dissection followed by radiotherapy.

Q. How will you reconstruct the large defect that has been surgically created in excising extensive lesion?

A. By pectoralis major flap.

(M) MALIGNANCY OROPHARYNX

Table 4.M-1: Oropharyngeal sites

A. Anterior wall	1. Posterior 1/3 of tongue
	2. Vallecula
B. Lateral wall	1. Tonsil
	2. Tonsillar fossa and faucial pillars
	3. Glossotonsillar sulci
C. Posterior wall	— Posterior pharyngeal wall
D. Superior wall	1. Inferior surface of soft palate
	2. Uvula

In general the staging of malignancy oropharynx is same as that of oral cavity (Table) the most common cases kept in examination are malignancy base tongue and malignancy tonsil. Three types of tissues are present in the oropharynx, viz.

1. Squamous cell lining giving rise to squamous cell corcinoma.

2. Lymphoid tissue (in palatine tonsils and lingual tonsils i.e. base of tongue) giving rise to non-hodgkins lymphoma.
3. Minor salivary glands (on soft palate, uvula and capsule of tonsil) giving rise to adenoid cystic carcinoma.

However since squamous cell carcinoma is the commonest malignancy encountered, further discussion would focus only on this type.

The lymph nodes that are most likely to get involved in malignancy of tonsil or base of tongue are level 2 (upper deep cervical or jugulodigastric) group of nodes.

Hence their palpation is must to complete the examination.

(N) MALIGNANCY TONGUE BASE (POSTERIOR 1/3RD)

Q. What is your diagnosis?

A. My diagnosis is (1) malignancy base tongue stage —— or (2) malignancy oropharynx stage —— (in case if extensive malignancy of tongue is involving other structures of oropharynx such as glossotonsillar sulcus, tonsil, tonsillar fossa, faucial pillars or vallaculae) or (3) malignancy base tongue (or oropharynx) stage —— extending to supraglottic larynx or (4) malignancy tongue stage —— (if the lesion has spread to anterior 2/3rd of tongue but is localized to the tongue only, and so on.

Q. Why do you say this is a malignancy?

A. The answer should be framed as described previously in malignancy of oral cavity taking into consideration the following points :

1. Age of patient.
2. Sex predilection.
3. Personal habits including the predisposing factors such as tobacco chewing, smoking, alcohol etc.
4. Symptoms (rapidly progressive non-healing lesion).
5. Signs on clinical examination suggestive of malignancy including appearance of lesion and spread.
6. Lymph node status being clinically significant (if applicable).

Q. What is the importance of palpation of tongue base during clinical staging?

A. Base of tongue should always be palpated because the lesion may deeply infiltrate and spread intramurally to the surrounding tongue substance, vallecular, epiglottis tonsillo- lingual sulcus, tonsils and supraglottic larynx. Hence the external inspection (indirect laryngoscopy) may just reveal a 'tip of iceberg' in some cases. Therefore palpation of base tongue is mandatory to clinically assess the extent of an infiltrative disease.

Q. What are the chances of lymph node metastasis in malignancy base tongue?

A. There are very high chances for malignancy of base tongue to give rise to cervical metastasis. Almost 2/3rd of patients present with cervical lymph node involvement. There is a likelihood of bilateral neck involvement since the lymphatics from base of tongue drain to bilateral jugolodigastric lymph nodes.

Note

Since the distant metastasis may occur in lungs and liver, it is mandatory to auscultate the chest and palpate the abdomen for organomegaly. Hence, the above points should be kept in mind when concluding clinical staging.

Q. How will you work up this case (or diagnose this case)?

A. Apart from routine examination such as HB, TLC, DLC, BT/ CT, ESR, X-ray chest (for secondary spread) a biopsy of the lesion is to be undertaken for histopathological evaluation to plan a definitive treatment.

Q. How will you treat the case?

A. I would like to treat this case by chemoradiotherapy (since most of the cases are of advanced stage and surgery as such is quite mutilating with poor post-operative results due to poor rehabilitation in our setup). The radiotherapy would encompass both the primary tumor as well as neck metastasis (if present).

Q. What are the surgical options for malignancy base tongue?

A. The surgical procedure to be adopted depends upon the extent of disease. For malignancy limited to tongue base, a total glossectomy with neck dissection is the treatment of choice. In case malignancy extends to lateral pharyngeal wall, then mandibulectomy along with total glossectomy, resection of lateral pharyngeal wall and neck dissection enbloc is the procedure of choice. If the malignancy extends to larynx then total glossectomy plus supraglottic laryngectomy along with neck dissection is the choiced procedure. All the surgical options should be followed by post-operative radiotherapy.

(O) MALIGNANCY TONSIL

Table 4.O-1: Spread of malignancy tonsil

1.	**LOCAL**	
(A)	Medially	- soft palate
		- tonsillar pillars
		- tonsillolingual sulcus
		- tongue
(b)	Superiorly	- soft palate
(c)	Laterally	- mandible
		- pterygoid muscles
		- parapharyngeal space
2.	**LYMPHATIC**	- jugulodigastric (level 2) lymph node
3.	**DISTANT**	- bone
		- lung
		- liver

Note

1. The involvement of mandible, retromolar trigone and pterygoid muscles lead to trismus.
2. The staging is to be done as per the table and should be accordingly discussed if asked.

Q. What is your diagnosis?

A. My diagnosis is (1) malignancy tonsil (if lesion is of the tonsils only) stage —— or (2) malignancy oropharynx (if lesion extends to surrounding areas) stage —— involving left (or right) tonsil, tonsillolingual sulcus, base tongue (accordingly include or exclude the sites involved).

Note

The status of lymph nodes if positive can always be described in the diagnosis although it is included in staging (some examiners always prefer to listen the status of lymph nodes separately).

Q. Why do you think it to be malignancy?

A. Same as that of malignancy tongue.

Note

Owing to infiltrative nature of malignant extension it is essential to palpate the disease in order to appreciate the occult induration and hence the extension. This is very important while staging the disease and planning out the treatment.

Q. What diagnostic work up should be undertaken in this patient?

A. Same as in malignancy tongue.

Q. Why do oral and oropharyngeal malignancies cause pain in the ear?

A. The earache in these cases is referred otalgia due to 2 mechanisms. Firstly, malignancy involving the tongue irritates the glossopharyngeal (IX) nerve and the sensations are carried along to tympanic branch of glossopharyngeal (or Jacobson's) nerve , thereby resulting in referred otalgia. Secondly the oropharyngeal malignancies can lead to irritation of the internal branch of superior laryngeal nerve (X). The sensations are carried through this to the auricular branch of vagus (Arnold's nerve) thereby resulting in referred otalgia.

Q. How will you treat an early (stage 1) carcinoma of tonsil?

A. An early lesion localized to tonsil is best treated by excision of the tonsil followed by RT both to the primary site as well as to the neck.

Q. How will you treat an advanced malignancy of tonsil (stage 3/4)?

A. The best treatment for an advanced oropharyngeal malignancy in terms of patient complains would be chemoradiation (since in most cases of advanced disease the surgery is mutilating with poor quality of life). The radiotherapy is to be focused on both the primary site and neck.

Q. What are the options of treating stage 2 disease?

A. In stage 2 disease, if the patient is a good surgical candidate a wide enbloc surgical resection involving lateral pharyngeal wall (including tonsil and fossa), hemimandibulectomy, glossectomy (if the tongue is involved) and neck dissection may be undertaken followed by curative R.T. Alternatively in case of poor surgical candidates chemoradiotherapy should be given.

Q. What is COMMANDO operation?

A. The word COMMANDO is an abbreviation of combined mandibulectomy, dissection of neck and oropharyngeal resection. This is undertaken for malignancies of lateral oropharyngeal wall including the tonsils.

(P) THYROGLOSSAL CYST

Q. What is your diagnosis?

A. My diagnosis is thyroglossal cyst.

Q. What is the etiology of thyroglossal cyst?

A. Embryologically thyroid gland descends from tongue into the neck along the thyroglossal tract that later on gets obliterated. If a cyst develops in the tract before obliteration, it is known as thyroglossal cyst.

Q. Why does it move with tongue protrusion?

A. Since thyroglossal tract is connected both to the tongue as well as to thyroid gland, the thyroglossal cyst moves up both on tongue protrusion as well as on deglutition.

Q. What additional diagnostic work up is needed to confirm the diagnosis?

A. The diagnosis is purely clinical and no further investigations are needed to confirm the diagnosis. However routine blood investigations for evaluating the preoperative status of patient is needed such as HB, TLC, DLC, BT, CT.

Q. How will you treat the case?

A. The treatment of choice is surgical excision by Sistrunk's operation.

Q. What is Sistrunk's operation?

A. In this operation the cyst along with the tract is removed and the part of hyoid between the lesser cornu with attached muscles is excised to prevent recurrence.

Note

1. If the patient presents with infected thyroglossal cyst, then antibiotics are to be given first till the infection is controlled only then the surgery is to be undertaken.
2. If infected thyroglossal cyst ruptures externally, this results in thryoglossal sinus which discharge mucus (in non-infective stage). In case of superadded infection the sinus discharges pus and is associated with tenderness with or without lymphadenopathy. A 'Sinugram' is undertaken to know the extent of the tract followed by Sistrunk's operation an a definitive treatment (Insert Figs. 4.P-1 & 4.P-2 about here).

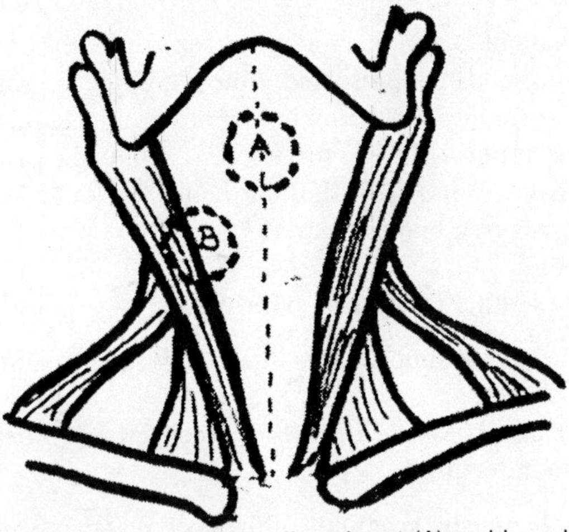

Fig. 4.P-1. Classical location of thyroglossal cyst (A) and branchial cyst (B).

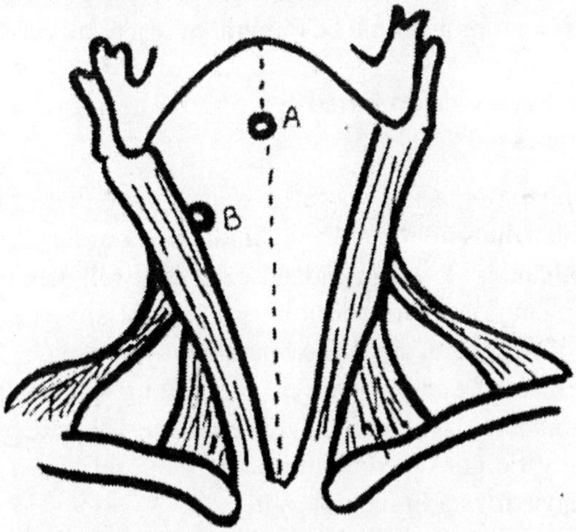

Fig. 4.P-2. Classical location of thyroglossal sinus (A) and branchial sinus (B).

(Q) BRANCHIAL CYST

Q. What is your diagnosis?

A. My diagnosis is a cystic swelling of neck and the first differential diagnosis that I would like to entertain is a branchial cyst.

Q. What are your points in favor of it being a branchial cyst?

A. The patient is a male (watch for sex) in its third decade (watch for age) and has presented with a gradually progressive neck swelling along the anterior border of sternomastoid at the junction of its upper 1/3rd & lower 2/3rd. This is firmly cystic in consistency and well defined hence I would like to make a diagnosis of a branchial cyst.

Q. Can a branchial cyst be painful?

A. Yes, in case of supperadded infection it can be painful and tender.

Q. What other possibilities in differential diagnosis would you like to entertain?

A. The other cystic swellings of the neck that can be thought of are lymphangioma and dermoid cyst (cystic degeneration in a lymph node or a tumor should be thought of in a relatively older patients.

Q. How have you excluded lymphangioma and a dermoid cyst in this case?

A. Lymphangioma is of a softer consistency than a branchial cyst and also does not have well demarcated borders. Dermoid on the other hand is very firm and tense and has well demarcated borders. Lymphangioma and dermoid can present anywhere in the upper part of neck. But since the branchial cyst is classically known to present at the upper part of neck along the anterior border of sternomastoid and owing to the characteristic site of presentation, firm cystic consistency and being well defined, I would like to diagnose it as a branchial cyst.

Q. Do you feel that it can be a cystic degeneration in a tumor or a lymph node?

A. Since this is a young healthy patient without any evidence of a primary malignancy or any malignant cachexia, the likelihood of such a possibility is minimal. The search for such a pathology may be undertaken if the histopathology of the cyst is suggestive of malignancy.

Q. How would you like to diagnose the case?

A. The diagnosis is mainly by clinical examination. However apart from routine investigations such as HB, TLC, DLC, BT/CT, ESR, and X-ray chest a fine needle aspiration cytology (FNAC) for confirming the diagnosis (and ruling out remote possibility of malignancy) may be undertaken.

Q. How will you treat the case?

A. The treatment of choice is surgical excision of the cyst along with its tract if present via a transverse incision along the cervical crease. Postoperatively the specimen is to be subjected to histopathological examination for ruling out malignancy.

Q. How does a branchial cyst arise?

A. There are various theories of origin. A branchial cyst may arise from branchial apparatus, or from thymopharyngeal duct or from inclusion of branchial epithelium into a lymph node. The latter theory is the most accepted.

Q. What is the characteristic of the fluid in branchial cyst?

A. The cyst contains straw coloured fluid with cholesterol crystals.

Note

1. In an infected branchial cyst a full course of antibiotic is given in the beginning to control infection. Only after the infection is controlled, surgical excision of the cyst is to be undertaken.
2. Branchial sinus (or fistula) is seen since birth at the junction of upper 1/3rd and lower 2/3rd of anterior border of sternomastoid. The theories of origin implicated are same as that of branchial cyst. The diagnosis is clinical plus supplemented by a sinogram to know the extent of sinus tract. The definitive treatment is surgical excision of the tract. In case of infected sinus, the infection is first controlled by antibiotics and then the operation is undertaken. Usually the tract goes up the tonsillar fossa and hence should be traced up and excised accordingly.

(R) RANULA

Q. What is your diagnosis?

A. My diagnosis is a benign cystic swelling in floor of mouth and I would like to entertain my first differential diagnosis as a ranula.

Q. What other differential diagnosis would you like to entertain?

A. The only other differential diagnosis for a benign cystic swelling in the floor of mouth would be a sublingual dermoid.

Q. What is a ranula

A. A ranula is a uni- or multilocular, mucus filled cyst in the floor of mouth. Ranula can be either simple or of plunging type.

Q. What is the difference between a simple ranula and a plunging ranula?

A. A simple ranula has an epithelial lining and is confined to the floor of mouth, while a plunging or burrowing ranula is lined by connective tissue (Not epithelium) and can extend into the neck. Do not target to do a bimanual palpation to rule out such an extension.

Q. Why do you say it is a ranula?

A. Since this is a young patient (watch for age) complaining of a chronic progressive swelling in the floor of mouth and on examination there is a typical bluish, translucent cyst on one side of frenulum, I would like to make a diagnosis of ranula.

Note

1. A ranula if gets repeatedly infected does not present as a typical bluish, translucent, smooth cyst, but rather a dull looking opaque cyst. Similar is the case with sublingual dermoid but the fluid in former is serous while in the latter, it is thick cheesy white material.
2. When there is a confusion in differentiating ranula with sublingual dermoid it is always safe to include two

differential diagnoses in your diagnosis, first one being ranula and second one being sublingual dermoid or the reverse as per the case.

3. Usually there is no significant lymphadenopathy in these 2 entities but still if the infection supervenes or otherwise, one can appreciate significant lymph nodes in neck (Fig. 4.R-1 about here).

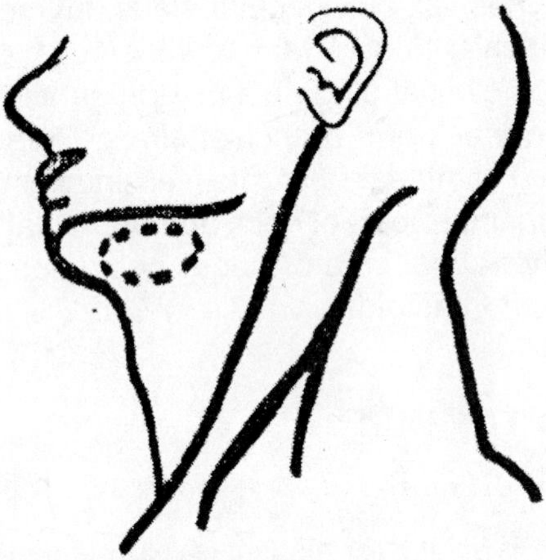

Fig. 4.R-1. Classical location of ranula.

Q. How will you investigate the case?

A. Since the diagnosis is mainly clinical, an aspiration of swelling may be undertaken to further confirm the diagnosis. Thc CT imaging has a role only if there is an extensive extension. However routine investigations such as Hb, TLC, DLC, BT/CT /ESR etc. need to be carried out as a part of preanaesthetic work up.

Q. How will you treat the case?

A. I would like to excise the cyst intraorally and include the sublingual gland if needed.

Note

A plunging ranula extending into the neck need to be marsupilized only along with excision of sublingual gland.

Q. Why do you want to excise sublingual gland?

A. If the gland is in close proximity to the cyst. I would like to excise it since these cysts are considered to arise from sublingual salivary gland according to one theory.

Note

The sinuses / fistula kept in the practical examination of ENT are only of 3 types viz. preauricular sinus, thyroglossal sinus / fistula and branchial sinus. Preauricular sinus presents in front of the ear, thyroglossal sinus usually presents in the midline in upper part of neck and branchial sinus. Preauricular sinus presents in front of the ear, thyroglossal sinus usually presents in the midline in upper part of neck and branchial sinus / fistula presents on the lateral side of upper neck along the anterior boarder of sternomastoid.

(S) PAROTID TUMOUR

Q. What is your diagnosis?

A. My diagnosis is benign (or malignant) parotid tumour.

Q. Why do you say that it is a parotid tumour?

A. The main reason of it being a parotid mass is because it is located in the parotid region and more importantly the ear lobule is shifted outwards and upwards.

Q. Why do you conclude it to be a benign tumour?

A. This is because this (middle-aged) patient has presented with a painless slow growing mass that is smooth (or lobulated), firm, non-tender and well-defined with normal overlying skin. Most important points in favour of benign lesion are the absence of facial nerve and lymph node involvement.

Q. When would you have called it malignant?

A. The mass should be suspected as being malignant if (i) the swelling is rapidly progressive, (ii) has become painful, (iii) facial nerve involvement is present, (iv) swelling is fixed to overlying skin and/or underlying structures (muscle viz. masseter and bone viz. mandible), (v) involvement of regional lymphnodes.

Q. What type of benign parotid tumour are you suspecting?

A. Pleomorphic adenoma because this is the most common benign tumor (that fits appropriately with the above description).

Q. How can you infer if superficial or deep lobe is involved?

A. The superficial lobe involvement (i.e. superficial to facial nerve) presents with a predominant swelling in the parotid region externally while the deep lobe involvement is predominantly characterized by a bulge in the lateral pharyngeal wall pushing the tonsil and tonsillar pillars medially. In the deep lobe tumour the external swelling is usually insignificant but the intraoral swelling is continuous with the external counterpart as confirmed by bimannual palpation.

Q. How will you differentiate this from parotid abscess?

A. Parotid abscess usually presents with acute pain and swelling associated with fever. The swelling is diffuse, extremely tender with pain of throbbing variety radiating to the ear and side of head. The skin overlying is hot, opening of Stenson's duct may show signs of inflammation / pus and level II lymph nodes may be enlarged / tender.

Q. How will you investigate the case?

A. Apart from routine investigation I would like to undertake a few special investigations such as CT & MRI (plain as well as contrast) – fine axial cuts of parotid and surrounding region. An ultrasound of neck would rule out the possibility of any significant lymphadenopathy. Most important the nature of the lesion needs to be confirmed by FNAC either as such or guided by imaging.

Q. How will you treat this patient?

A. Superficial parotidectomy under general anaesthesia.

Q. How will you treat malignant parotid tumour?

A. Total radical parotidectomy with sacrifice of facial nerve only if the malignancy is localized within the parotid gland and is ressectable.

Q. How will you treat a deep-lobe parotid tumour?

A. Total conservative parotidectomy with preservation of facial nerve.

Q. What are the complications of parotidectomy?

A. Hematoma, facial weakness or iatrogenic palsy, local anesthesia, salivary fistula formation, gustatory sweating (Frey's syndrome).

Q. What is the role of RT in management of parotid tumour?

A. Radiotherapy may be given in case of malignant tumour or in massive benign tumour where there is a doubtful involvement of facial nerve following surgery (proved on frozen section).

Q. What other conditions can you think apart from benign parotid tumour.

A. Chronic sialadenitis and sialolithiasis, granulomatious diseases such as tuberculosis, sarcoidosis (uveo-parotid fever or Heerford's syndrome), actinomycosis, vascular malformations (venous, lymphatic), traumatic pseudocyst, lipoma, masseter hypertrophy.

Q. Is it possible to ressect the underlying mandible along with malignancy if it is involved?

A. In case the malignant tumour is fixed to underlying bone, it can be ressected en-bloc along with involved masseter, provided the pathology can be radically cleared.

(T) THYROID SWELLING

Q. What is your diagnosis?

A. Thyroid swelling.

Q. Why it is a thyroid swelling?

A. Because it moves with deglutition and is in the region of thyroid gland.

Q. How can you comment upon the functional status of thyroid gland?

A. Functionally the patient seems to be euthyroid as he does not seem to have any symptoms suggestive of hypo- or hyper-thyroidism.

Note

If there are symptoms suggestive of hyper- or hypothyroidism, that have to be commented upon in detail.

Q. What are the symptoms of hypothyroidism?

A. Apart from generalized symptoms (weakness, fatigue, cold-intolerance, weight gain, hair-loss, edema of hands and face, dry thick skin and hair, decreased sweating) the otolaryngological symptoms include deafness, tinnitus, imbalance, speech alterations, enlarged tongue and middle ear effusion. The cardiovascular symptoms include bradicardia, mild increase in blood pressure and peripheral oedema while gastrointestinal manifestations include anorexia, intermittent nausea / vomiting, constipation, dysphagia and bloating sensation. Tracheal compression would result in shortness of breath. Headache, somnolence in daytime with insomnia at night, physical and mental slowing, decreased reflexes, depression and anxiety would characterize central nervous system involvement. Joint-stiffness, bone-pains muscle cramps and weakness are not uncommon.

Q. What are the main features of hyperthyroidism?

A. Apart from general symptoms (palpitations / increased pulse rate, fatigue, irritability, weight loss, heat-intolerance, anxiety and tendency to increase in bowel movements) the signs would include tachycardia, warm and moist skin, fine tremors of fingers (on extension), exophthalmos, eyelid retraction, lid-lag and occasional arrhythmias. (**NOTE**: Thyroid gland is usually enlarged and the features of surrounding compression if present should be noted and mentioned).

Final Note

In case the above symptoms of hypothyroidism or hyperthyroidism are seen the diagnosis is made as "***Thyroid swelling with hypo- (or hyper-) thyroidism***".

Q. What are the features suggestive of malignancy of thyroid.

A. A malignant tumour is likely to be extrathyroidal, with fixation to underlying soft tissue (no effect of swallowing). It is more likely to blend with surroundings and result in decreased parotid pulsations due to displacement / compression of carotids. Dysphagia may occur due to oesophageal compression, while Horner's syndrome may point towards cervical sympathetic involvement. Compression of trachea may result in wheezing dyspnoea in supine position, while its invasion may give rise to hemoptysis. Similarly recurrent laryngeal nerve involvement as well as laryngeal invasion may cause hoarseness. Most important is the involvement of cervical lymph node (significantly enlarged and tender).

Q. Can a large benign thyroid swelling be confused with malignancy?

A. A large goiter is known to displace trachea, reduce carotid pulsations and cause dysphagia. However if carefully assessed the differentiation can be easily made.

Q. What are the causes of sudden increase in size of thyroid gland?

A. Infection haemorrhage and malignancy.

Q. How will you differentiate between benign and malignant thyroid swelling?

A. The 2 most important investigations needed for this purpose are ultrasound and FNAC. The US would localize the single / isolated vs. multicentric and cystic vs. solid lesions as well as reveal any cervical lymphadenopathy. FNAC is known to be the most important single investigation to differentiate benign from malignant lesion through cytology. In addition thyroid-binding-globulin (TBG) in blood acts as a very sensitive marker of extent of disease. Chest X-ray can help finding a pulmonary metastases.

Q. What is the role of thyroid scan in the primary diagnosis?

A. I-123 scan usually results in a cold nodule signifying malignancy while a hot-nodule signifies a toxic adenoma. On the contrary the Selenium-scan reveals a hot-nodule in malignancy since the malignant tissue actively takes up the selenium. However the role of scan is just supportive and is not undertaken as the first step.

Q. How will you assess the functional status of thyroid?

A. The single most important investigation is measurement of serum TSH. This, if found elevated, signifies hypothyroidism while if decreased suggests hyperthyroidism.
(NOTE: For combined assessment of T3, T4, TSH refer to a textbook).

Q. How will you manage hypothyroidism?

A. Thyroxine hormone supplementation (eltroxin) orally with dose adjusted as per the blood hormone profile and clinical performance. In addition iodine supplementation and use of iodized salt should be undertaken.

Q. How will you manage hyperthyroidism?

A. A toxic nodule causing problematic symptoms may be excised surgically. The medical management usually consists of antithyroid drugs—the important ones are methimazole and propyl-thio-uracil. The effect of treatment is titrated with the clinical symptoms and blood hormone profile.

Q. What type of malignancy is seen in thyroid gland?

A. Well-differentiated cancers are the most common ones encountered, viz., papillary and follicular. (See Table p. 61).

Q. How will you differentiate the well-differentiated cancers with medullary cancer.

A. Medullary cancer of thyroid is characterized by increased levels of serotonin (flushing, headache, breathlessness, sweating, fainting), protaglandins and histaminase (concentration directly proportional to metastatic disease). The blood chemistry reveals increased calcium, increased calcitonin, 5-HT, and VMA, while urinary examination reveals increased 5-HIAA & 24-hr catecholamines.

Q. What are the types of undifferentiated malignancies encountered?

A. Medullary and anaplastic cancer.

Q. How will you manage well-differentiated thyroid cancer?

A. Total thyroidectomy with neck dissection is undertaken in case of resectable disease followed by radioactive I^{123}-therapy to take care of occult disease. In unressectable pathology radioactive I^{123} with or without external beam radiotherapy is preferred.

Q. What is the difference between hemithyroidectomy, near-total thyroidectomy, total thyroidectomy and completion thyroidectomy?

A. Hemithyroidectomy with or without isthmusectomy undertaken for a solitary nodule with or without involvement of isthmus. Near-total thyroidectomy is done in extensive benign thyroid disease e.g. goiter : here a small rim of normal thyroid gland is preserved to retain the bare minimal endocrine functions. Total thyroidectomy refers to radical thyroid excision specially in case of malignancy. Completion thyroidectomy refers to removal of residual thyroid tissue from previous thyroid surgery.

Q. What is the prognosis of thyroid cancer?

A. Papillary cancer carries an excellent prognosis followed by follicular cancer. Medullary cancer carries a bad prognosis anaplastic cancer is the worst of all.

TABLE: COMPARISON OF PAPILLARY AND FOLLICULAR THYROID CANCER

Features	Papillary	Follicular
1. Age and sex	Young female; 40 yr	Old female; 50 yr
2. Predisposing factors	Irradiation	Endemic goitre
3. Incidence	Most common	Second common
4. Prognosis	Best	-
5. Capsule	Pseudocapsule; Late invasion	True capsule; Early invasion
6. Lymphatic spread	Common	-
7. Blood-borne spread	-	Common
8. Pulmonary metastasis	Uncommon (military infiltrates)	Common (multiple large rounded shadows)
9. Osteolytic lesions	Uncommon	Seen with bone pains

(U) BELLS PALSY

Q. What is your diagnosis?

A. Idiopathic facial palsy or the Bells palsy

Q. Why do you say so? OR why do you call it as idiopathic Bells palsy?

A. I say so because the patient has presented with unilateral facial palsy of acute onset and I have excluded all the major causes of unilateral facial involvement.

Q. What are the causes that you have excluded?

A. I could not find any evidences of otitis media or tumours of middle ear such as glomus, tympanomastoid malignancy or any lymphadenopathy. There is no history of either facial / parotid trauma or any operative intervention. Similarly I have excluded the possibilities of multiple sclerosis, poliomyelitis, basal meningitis, infective polyneuritis and systemic diseases like diabetes mellitus and hypothyroidism on the basis of history and clinical examination. Therefore I feel that this condition is idiopathic.

Q. What is known about the etiology of Bells palsy? OR why does Bells palsy occur?

A. Bells palsy is thought to follow some sort of viral infection such as herpes simplex, herpes zoster, EBV; or is a consequence to vascular ischemia due to stress and cold primarily or due to exudation inside the nerve sheath secondary to inflammation leading to compromised microvascular circulation. Lately it has been hypothesized that Bells palsy may be a sort of autoimmune disorder. In general the exact etiology is still not established.

Q. What are the clinical symptoms apart from the facial asymmetry that need due attention?

A. The other important clinical features are epiphora, noise intolerance (stapedial paralysis), loss of taste (involvement of cauda tympani nerve), and otalgia.

Q. How will you investigate this case?

A. Apart from routine investigations like Hb, TLC, DLC, BT/CT, PT/PC, ESR/ PCV etc., I would like to do some topognostic tests to establish the site of nerve involvement. Moreover I would definitely like to undertake the nerve-excitability testing thrice a week to monitor nerve degeneration by comparing it with the normal side.

Q. What are the topognostic tests?

A. Schirmer's test (or lacrimation test), salivary flow test, topical subjective gustometry and stapedial reflex.

Q. What will be the status of hearing impairment in this case?

A. The hearing will be absolutely normal.

Q. How will you treat this case?

A. Since this condition is mostly reversible, the first step would be to reassure the patient of the outcome. Secondly no treatment is required in case of incomplete paralysis. However analgesics may be given to combat pain and eye care (with artificial tears) should be instituted properly. In case of complete paralysis oral steroids (prednisolone) should be given for a week and the recovery assessed by electrodiagnostic tests. Apart from this the patient may be given vasodilators, multivitamins, electrical stimulation of facial muscles and local physiotherapy as a part of treatment protocol.

Q. What is the role of surgery?

A. The role of surgery is controversial. This is carried out with an aim to decompress the nerve in order to enhance the microcirculation. The main indication is when ENG demonstrates 70-90% degeneration within 2 weeks after onset of bells palsy. (NOTE: Surgery is not advisable after 2 weeks since viral illness has resolved and early regeneration has begun.

Q. What surgery is undertaken?

A. The is carried out with an aim to decompress the facial nerve in order to enhance the microcirculation. Although transmastoid decompression has been reported for decompression of vertical segments, the current protocol involves decompression of meatal and labyrinthine segments through middle cranial fossa approach.

Q. What is the prognosis of Bells palsy?

A. More than 80% have full recovery and around 15% show partial recovery with some residual dysfunction. Those with recurrent paralysis are more likely to show some residual deficits.

5

Differential Diagnoses

I. NECK MASS

Remember the mnemonic 'KITENS' for a patient complaining of a neck mass

K **Congenital** or developmental (branchial cyst, thyroglossal cyst, sebaceous cyst, dermoid cyst, hemangioma, lymphangioma, laryngocele, pharyngocele or diverticulum, thymic swelling, ectopic thyroid tissue).

I **Inflammatory or infective**

(a) Lymphadentis—bacterial including pyogenic and tubercular, viral, granulomatous, fungal actinomycosis.

(b) Generalized swelling of floor of mouth extending to neck spaces : Ludwig's angina.

T **Traumatic:** hematoma with or without infection.

E **Endocrinal causes:** Thyroid, parathyroid or carotid body tumor

N **Neoplasm:**

(a) primary : Lymphoma thyroid, salivary gland, lipoma, rhabdomyosarcoma, nerve sheath tumor.

(b) secondaries :

1. from squamous or occult primary in head and neck region or
2. from distant primary such as prostrate, uterus, breast, lung, intestine and kidney (remember the 'PUBLIK')

S **Systematic** - psychiatric such as globus hystericus.

CLINICAL FEATURES OF SOME ENTITIES PRESENTING AS NECK MASS

(A) Cystic hygroma

1. Child (or infant) presenting with painless and slowly progressive swelling in the neck since birth.

2. The site of the swelling is usually in lower 1/3rd (posterior triangle) of neck or axilla / cheek, lobulated, softly cystic, non-tender (tender if infected), partially compressible, diffuse edges and ill defined.
3. Classically it is brilliantly transilluminant but is not always so.
4. Increases in size with coughing and crying.

(B) Carotid body tumor

1. Middle aged person presenting as a slowly progressive swelling on the lateral aspect of neck, at the upper border of thyroid cartilage.
2. swelling characteristics are its being smooth or lobulated and non-tender.
3. The swelling can be moved from side to side but not along the axis of great vessels of neck.
4. Carotid pulsations are transmitted on the careful inspection (and palpation).

(C) Sternomastoid tumor

1. A young child (or infant) presenting with a neck swelling in the sternomastoid muscle along its anterior boarder.
2. The swelling is usually small, oblong in shape with its long axis in the length of the sternomastoid muscle.
3. The consistency is firm and swelling is well defined.
4. The patient may present with apparent toricollis also.

(D) Ludwig's angina

1. Sudden onset of pain and swelling in upper part of neck usually with marked prostration and fever.
2. Marked swelling of the floor of mouth including tongue.
3. Inability to close the mouth fully associated with dribbling of salvia and inability to feed normally.
4. On examination: red, hot, tender, tense and indurated swelling in submandibular region and floor of mouth.
5. The swelling may compress the airway tract leading to partial respiratory obstruction.

II. SWELLING IN FLOOR OF MOUTH

1. Dermoid cyst
2. Ranula and plunging ranula presenting as a neck swelling
3. Ludwig's angina
4. Traumatic hematoma
5. Malignancy

III. NECK SWELLING INCREASING IN SIZE ON VALSALVA

1. Laryngocele
2. Pharyngocele
3. Venous phlebectasia.

6

Instruments for E.N.T. Examinations and Operations

Undergraduates in E.N.T should have basic knowledge about the instruments commonly used in E.N.T examinations (used in OPD) and operations (used in OT). The student should also know the various indications and basic steps of operation in which that particular instrument is used.

I. GENERAL EXAMINATION SET USED IN OPD

1. Head Mirror

Head mirror with adjustable head-band consists of a concave mirror 9.0 diameter with a central hole (about 2.0 cm) and a head-band.

Indications

Indications in examination and minor procedures of the ear, nose and throat by reflecting light from a light source.

2. Thudicum nasal speculum

Indication

1. *Diagnostic* : for anterior rhinoscopy i.e examination of anterior part of nasal cavity. The structures seen are: vestibule; anterior part of the nasal septum; anterior part of the inferior and middle turbinates; any pathological lesion if present can be visualized.
2. *Therapeutic*: used in F.B extraction, antral puncture, polypectomy, S.M.R. and septoplasty operations etc.

3. Lack's tongue depressor

Indications

1. Examination of the vestibule, oral cavity, floor of mouth, oral tongue, hard & soft palate, and oropharynx.
2. In posterior rhinoscopy along with posterior rhinoscopy mirror.
2. Minor operations: peritonsillar abscess drainage, biopsy from oral cavity / oropharynx.
3. Can be used for retraction of cheek and lip in internal operations.

4. Indirect laryngoscopic mirror:

Indications: in indirect laryngoscopy

1. *Diagnostic :* to visualize and detect any pathology of the base of the tongue, valleculla, glosso-epiglottic fold, epiglottis, pharyngo-epiglottic folds, ary epiglottic folds, arytenoids, inter-arytenoid region, pyriform sinus, inlet of the larynx, supraglottic region, ventricular bands, vocal cords, anterior and posterior commissures, subglottis and first few rings of the trachea.
2. *Therapeutic :*
   - to assist removal of penetrating foreign body (e.g. fish bone) from tonsil, tonsillolingual sulcus, the base of tongue, valleculae, pyriform fossa.
   - to assist in taking biopsy from the larynx and hypopharynx.

5. Posterior rhinoscopy mirror

Posterior rhinoscopy mirror is used in posterior rhinoscopy.

Indications :

1. *diagnostic*: used in examination of posterior part of the nasal cavity and nasopharynx. The structures seen are: anteriorly: choanal apertures, posterior end of the nasal septum, posterior part of the nasal cavities, posterior end of the inferior turbinates and meati, roof of nasopharynx and adenoids (in children); laterally: Eustachian tube openings, tubal eminence, fossa of Rossenmuller and lateral nasopharyngeal wall; inferiorly: superior surface of the soft palate.

6. Nasal packing forceps

Indications

It is used in all nasal operations for:

1. Removal of foreign bodies and bone chips etc .
2. Nasal packing, cleaning of crusts, etc
3. Removal of spicule like foreign body such as fish bone from orophaynx and oral cavity.

7. Eustachian catheter (Metallic)

Indications:

1. *Diagnostic*: to assess the Eustachian tube patency by catheterisation, using politzer bag in combination with Eustachian tube catheter.
2. *Therapeutic :*
   (a) to inflate the middle ear and the blocked Eustachian tube.
   (b) often used in removal of foreign body of the nose.
   (c) sometimes used as suction cannula.

EUSTACHIAN TUBE CATHETERISATION

Instruments used

1. Eustachian catheter
2. Politzer bag with adjustable adapter.

Technique: the nasal cavity is sprayed with local anaesthetic (10% xylocaine) and the catheter is passed along the floor till the tip (facing down) has reached the posterior nasopharyngeal wall. It is then withdrawn a little and turned (alternately medially and laterally) 90 degree when it slips into the Eustachian tube opening. The catheter is then connected with politzer bag and the air is pushed into the catheter by pumping politzer bag and making entry of air through the Eustachian tube up to the middle ear. The patient is simultaneously asked if he can appreciate the ear air insufflation.

8. Aural speculum

The pinna is to be pulled upwards, backward and outward in adult and outward and downward in children to make the canal straight to facilitate insertion of speculum.

Indications:

1. *Diagnostic* (otoscopy):
   (a) For examination of the external canal and tympanic membrane.
   (b) can be fitted with Siegle's pneumatic system for visualization of tympanic membrane mobility.
2. *Therapeutic:*
   (a) Aural cleaning through a speculum.
   (b) Assist in removal of wax, F.B. etc.
   (c) Used in myringotomy, stapedectomy, myringoplasty.

9. Otoscope

Indications :

Indications examination of the external canal and tympanic membrane.

Advantages: Enables magnified view of the drum and external canal. Being battery operated, examination can be carried out in situations of a power failure.

10. Jobson Horne's probe with ring curette:

Indications :

1. Serrated probe end is used as cotton swab carrier to clean aural discharge.
   (a) Curette can be used to remove wax, foreign body, and granulation.

11. Aural syringe

Indications :

Removal of foreign body and wax by syringing.

Technique of syringing: this is done in sitting position with a kidney-tray approximately at the subauricular position. Sterile water jet and the at body temp (37 degree C) is directed posterosuperiorly and the washed material is collected in the tray.

Complications:

1. Vaso-vagal syncope
2. Tympanic membrane rupture

3. Injury of the external canal and otitis externa
4. Labyrinthine stimulation and vertigo.

Contraindications

Otitis externa and otitis media.

12. Tuning forks

For hearing assessment by Rinne, Weber and ABC methods the commonly used tuning forks are of 256, 512, 1024 Hz but that of 512 Hz is most useful as the intensity of sound is long lasting.

Indications :

Diagnosis of different types of deafness viz. conductive, sensorineural and the mixed.

13. Siegle's pneumatic speculum

Indications :

1. Gives magnified view of the aural pathology and shows mobility of the tympanic membrane.
2. Used in fistula test.

II. TONSILLECTOMY SET

14. Guillotine

Guillotine was used in guillotine method of tonsillectomy operation and is now outdated.

15. Boyle Davis mouth gag

It has two parts :
1. Tongue blade
2. Jaw piece : retracts the upper jaw teeth.

Indications :

1. In dissection method of tonsillectomy
2. Surgery of the palate and the nasopharynx
3. Adenoidectomy.

16. **Tonsil holding forceps (Denis Browne)** is used to hold and to pull the tonsil medially during tonsillectomy. This will help to stretch the anterior pillar before incision and also to separate tonsil during dissection.
17. **Waugh's long dissecting forceps** is used during dissection of the tonsil, it can be used in catching bleeding points and putting in swabs.
18. **Anterior pillar retractor with dissector**: The retractor end retracts the anterior tonsillar pillar after the tonsillectomy and, the tonsillar fossa from its bed is visualized for any bleeding point or residual tonsillar tissue. The dissector end is used for dissection of tonsils.
19. **Eve's Tonsil snare with wire** is used to crush and detach lower pole of the tonsil in the final stage of delivery of tonsil.
20. **Tonsillar artery forceps** for grasping bleeding vessels of tonsillar fossa for hemostasis during and after tonsillectomy. This is long for better view of tonsillar bed while working at a depth.
21. **Ligature slipper or knot tier** helps to slip the ligature over the tip of forceps during ligation of bleeding point of the tonsillar bed following tonsillectomy operation.

III. INSTRUMENTS FOR OTHER OPERATIONS IN THROAT

22. **Quinse or peritonsillar abscess forceps** acts both as knife for incision and forceps to dilate the incision in cases of peritonsillar abscess drainage.
23. **St. Clair Thomson adenoid curette with cage** is used in adenoidectomy operation. The instrument is held in dagger-holding position and is passed behind soft palate keeping in midline. The adenoid are curetted with a sweep and is held by the cage to prevent from spillage either in the nasopharynx or larynx. Care must be taken while curretting to prevent injury to the eustachian tube opening which may lead to tubal stenosis (and middle ear disease). Incomplete curretting results in adenoid remnants that may lead to reactionary hemorrhage.

24. **Doyne's mouth gag** is used to open the mouth for anteriorly based intra-oral surgery.
25. **Fergeuson's mouth gag** is used to open the mouth in cases of minimal trismus for intra-oral surgery.
26. **Yaunkauer's nasopharyngoscope**: In cases where indirect mirror examination of nasopharynx is not possible this is a good alternative for direct examination of the nasopharynx and in obtaining biopsy from suspicious lesions.
27. **Direct laryngoscope**: Direct laryngoscope has 3 parts (1) Blade that goes inside the larynx and is attached to the (2) Handle (3) Proximal light source either battery operated bulbs (seen in older models, but now uncommonly used) or fiber optic cable connected to a cold light source (seen in modern models). *Grasped by a single hand with thumb on the thumb rest and the instrument is gently introduced after making a proper position of the patient (flexion of neck and extension at atlanto-occipital joint). Care is taken to avoid injury to lips and base of tongue during insertion. Epiglottis is lifted and the laryngeal inlet is analyzed by firmly lifting the neck. Care is to be taken to avoid lever action on incisors (as fulcrum) or else damage of teeth would result.*

Indications :

1. *Diagnostic:* To visualize the larynx if mirror examination fails as commonly happens in overhanging epiglottis.
   (a) To assess the cause of respiratory distress in children / infants such as laryngeal edema, diphtheria, foreign body etc.
   (b) To completely assess the extent of tumor involvement of larynx and to take a biopsy from suspicions site.
   (c) To differentiate between vocal cord paralysis and fixity by probing the arytenoids.

2. *Therapeutic:*
   (a) For endotracheal intubation.
   (b) Removal of foreign body

28. Oesophagoscope

Small handle with long lumen tube (blade) that is calibrated so as to know the length of insertion during oesophagoscopy. The lighting system is same as in a direct laryngoscope.

Indications :

1. *Diagnostic:* To assess the site of obstruction in case of:
   (a) Malignancy or
   (b) Corrosive / benign stricture
   (c) To obtain biopsy from suspicious site etc.
2. *Therapeutic:*
   (a) To remove an impacted foreign body.
   (b) To dilate a stricture.
   (c) To introduce a nasogastric tube or MB tube in case or malignancy with compromised lumen.

29. Bronchoscope

Small handle with a long lumen tube that has multiple openings at the distal end and an additional portal for oxygenation at proximal end. The distal openings facilitate the aeration of contralateral bronchus during bronchoscopy.

Indications:

1. *Diagnostic:*
   (a) To confirm a doubtful diagnosis of a foreign body in airway tract.
   (a) To assess the site of bleeding in cases presenting with hemoptysis.
   (a) To obtain biopsy from the suspicious site.
2. *Therapeutic:*
   (a) To extract an impacted foreign body.
   (a) To excise small polypoidal growth in airway tract.

Note

1. The size of bronchoscope varies with age. In infants and and small children a size of 1 is preferred. In a large child a size of 6 to 7 is used while for an adult a size 8 to 9 is appropriate.

2. As far as possible a large size is used (for better oxygenation, better visualization and better manipulation) but care is to be taken that the size is not too large to cause damage of airway tract mucosa.
3. Negus type of osophagoscope consists of proximal illumination while Jackson type of oesophagoscope has distal illumination. The size of oesophagoscope to be used in children is 10 mm × 25 mm while that of adult is 16 mm × 45 mm.

ASSOCIATED INSTRUMENTS

Crocodile action grasping forceps

Used along with bronchoscope, oesophagoscope and direct laryngoscope to extract a foreign body. Available in different sizes.

Crocodile action cupped (biopsy) forceps

Used along with bronchoscope, esophagoscope and direct laryngoscope to obtain a biopsy. Available in different sizes.

IV. INSTRUMENTS USED IN VARIOUS NASAL OPERATIONS

30. Lichtwitz trocar and cannula

Indications :

1. *Diagnostic*:
   (a) to confirm the presence of pus in the maxillary sinus (proof puncture) and to establish the diagnosis of maxillary sinusitis.
   (b) cytological examination of antral wash out fluid.
2. *Therapeutic:* to drain out pus in acute maxillary sinusitis the maxillary antrum is punctured through inferior meatus, usually under local anaesthesia.

31. Muco-perichondrial elevator

1. Killian's type.
2. Free elevator.

Indications

Used for separating and elevating muco-perichondrial flaps in S.M.R or septoplasty operation.

32. St. Clair Thomson's nasal speculum (long bladed)

Indications

In S.M.R operation after elevating of muco-perichondrail flaps on both sides, the blades are engaged as such to keep the two separated flaps apart, so that while manipulating the cartilage the chances of tearing the flaps can be minimized, otherwise there is a risk of septal perforation.

33. Killian's nasal speculum (long bladed)

Indications :

1. Same as St. Clair Thomson's nasal speculum in S.M.R or septoplasty operation and also.
2. In polypectomy operation, the blades are used to retract medial and lateral walls arround the polyp so as to better visualize the polyp and avoid injury to surrounding during polypectomy. Also the blades can be adjusted and fixed with screw during the operation with less strain on the assistant's hand holding the instrument.

34. Killian's Bayonet-shaped nasal gouge

Indications :

Used along with mallet in S.M.R operation to remove the maxillary crest and septal spur after separation of mucoperichondrial flaps.

35. Luc forceps

Indications :

1. In nasal operations: S.M.R., septoplasty, and Caldwell Luc operation to remove bone, cartilage and soft tissue.
2. In transnasal polypectomy for holding and avulsing the polyp.
3. Can be used to take punch biopsies from nasal cavity, nasopharynx and oropharynx.

36. Ballenger's swivel knife

It is known as swivel since the cutting blades revolve around two bars.

Indications :

In S.M.R operation to excise the septal cartilage after elevation of mucoperichondrial flaps.

37. Glegg's nasal snare

Indication :

In nasal polypectomy the pedicle of the polyp is held by snare and the polyp is avulsed.

38. Higginson's syringe

It is used with Lichtwitz cannula to lavage maxillary sinus. It consists of a rubber tube with adapter for cannula at one end, a central pouching and a one-way valve at the other end to facilitate unidirectional flows towards the adapter end. A negative pressure in the central pouching draws water inside from one end and a positive pressure created by pressing the central pouch pushes the water jet towards the adapter end (hence into the cannula / maxillary sinus).

34. Walsham forceps and Asche's forceps

Indications :

In reduction of fracture of the nasal bones (Walsham forceps) and that of fracture of nasal septum (Asche's forceps).

V. INSTRUMENTS USED IN VARIOUS OPERATIONS OF THE EAR

39. Bone gouge

Indications :

1. Removal of cortical mastoid bone chips in mastoid operations with the help of a mallet. Wider gouge is safer. The gouge should be used parallel to the structures to be exposed.

2. Can also be used in Caldwell Luc operation, S.M.R.

40. Chisel

Chisel is used for lowering the facial bridge in radical mastoidectomy.

41. Lampert's curette

Indications :

1. In different types of mastoidectomies to curette diseased mastoid air-cells and granulation tissue and to
2. Curette anterior and posterior buttress after breaking the bridge.

42. Electric drill

Electric drill is used to drill mastoid bone in different mastoid operations. It is a better alternative of bone gouge and facilitates quicker work and also reduces the chance of damage to facial nerve. It can also be used in middle ear operations to work on foot plate and ossicles.

43. Myringotomy knife

Indications :

For giving a neck incision in tympanic membrane bulge during myringotomy operation in acute otitis media etc

44. Aditus seeker with curette

Indications :

During a mastoidectomy operation the seeker helps to identify the aditus-ad-antrum in case of doubt while, the curette part is used to scoop the diseased air-cells.

45. Aural snare

Indication :

It is used to remove aural polyp of the middle ear via the external canal. To avoid injury to the facial nerve and ossicles, the snare must be passed smoothly and clamped across the pedicle instead of avulsing it.

46. Burr points / Drill bits

These are either of cutting type or of polishing type. Both are used along with a electric drill machine for cutting or polishing a bony cavity. Available in different sizes and shapes as per the utility. In an undergraduate examination usually a round cutting (serrated) burr point is asked. This is usually made up of tungsten carbide. However a diamond drill bit (without serration) can also be asked.

A large size cutting burr point facilitates faster cutting while a diamond burr point is usually preferred in critical situations where there is a danger of damaging a vital structure underneath the bone. With a diamond burr point the time consumed in surgery is more but the safety factor is enhanced as compared to a cutting drill bit.

47. Mallet

Mallet or hammer is made up of alloy and is used along with gouge, chisel and osteotome in the bone work (cutting, slicing, remodeling) during operations of ear, nose and paranasal sinuses.

48. Mollison's self retaining, haemostatic post aural retractor

1. Primarily during mastoidectomy to retract the skin so as to expose the underlying bone after a post-aural incision.
2. Can also be used to retract the incised edges of skin during lateral rhinotomy incision.
3. Can also retract the cartilaginous ends of thyroid lamina during laying of tissue.

49. Endaural Retractor

Primarily used during mastoidectomy to retract the cartilaginous framework of pinna for a wide exposure of the underlying bone after an end aural incision. The blade used along with it retracts the temporalis muscle. Other uses are same as with Mollison's postaural retractor.

50. Self retaining ear speculum

Used during endomeatal ear surgery to widen the exposure for better manipulation.

VI. TRACHEOSTOMY

Indications :

1. **Obstructive indications:** (1) advanced laryngeal cancer; (2) diphtheretic laryngitis; (3) oedema larynx; (4) F.B larynx; (5) laryngeal papillomatosis in children (6) other causes of laryngeal stridor; etc.
2. **Non-obstructive indications:** (1) head injury; (2) comatose patient; (3) barbiturate and other poisonings; (4) assisted ventilation for respiratory depression; etc.

51. Tracheostomy tube (metal)

Consists of outer tube and inner tube; inner tube is longer than the outer so that when the tube gets blocked, on removal of the inner tube the blockage is cleared.

Varieties

1. **Fuller's bi-valve type**: bi-valve helps in introduction into tracheostome (acts as a dilator). The opening on the posterosuperior wall of the inner tube helps in decannulation i.e determines whether normal air passage is established on blocking the tracheostomy stoma.
2. **Jackson type**: movable shield with pilot.

Note

Speaking valve is now available with inner tube for a tracheostomised patient to speak. Patient can talk without closing the outer opening with finger. This is one of the various procedures of speech rehabilitation in a laryngectomised patient.

52. Portex tracheostomy tube (plastic)

Single tube, no inner tube, available in non-cuffed and cuffed varieties. Non-cuffed variety is commonly used whereas the cuffed variety is suitable when the tube is connected to the respirator in cases of assisted ventilation to avoid air-leak.

53. Romsons Tracheostomy tube

This is made of plastic material and is a cheap alternative to portex tracheostomy tube. A disadvantage uncommonly encountered with this tube is that sometimes its collar gets detached from the tubular part dislodging the latter into the trachea.

54. Tracheal dilator

Helps to introduce the tracheostomy tube by retracting the tracheostome edges.

55. Double hook retractor

Is used to retract skin, superficial and deep fascia, and muscles of the neck across the incision line during exposure of the trachea.

56. Single hook (sharp) retractor

Is used to fix the larynx by retracting the cricoid cartilage prior to tracheal incision during tracheostomy operation.

57. Single hook (blunt) retractor

Is used for retracting the isthmus of thyroid gland or other tissues for exposure of tracheal wall in mid or low tracheostomy operation.

VII. NASAL ENDOSCOPY

58. Nasal endoscope

This is a rigid, fibre optic illuminated, Hopkin rod telescope for in depth diagnosis and treatment of sinunasal diseases. It is used for sinunasoscopy along with a fiber optic cable and a cold light source.

Indications :

1. Diagnostic: To inspect nasal cavity in
   (a) Chronic sinusits.
   (b) Suspected malignancy
   (c) Repeated epistaxis where the cause cannot be seen.
   (d) CSF rhinorrhoea suspicion.

   Also used to inspect nasopharynx for occult malignancy.
2. *Therapeutic :*
   1. Functional endoscopic sinus surgery (FESS).
   2. To obtain biopsy from posterior part of nasal cavity or nasopharynx.

3. Periodic examination of a closed cavity (sinus or nasal cavity or nasopharynx) for recurrence of disease after operation.

59. Blacklesley nasal forceps

Usually used with nasal endoscope to obtain biopsy or in FESS. It can be straight or angulated.

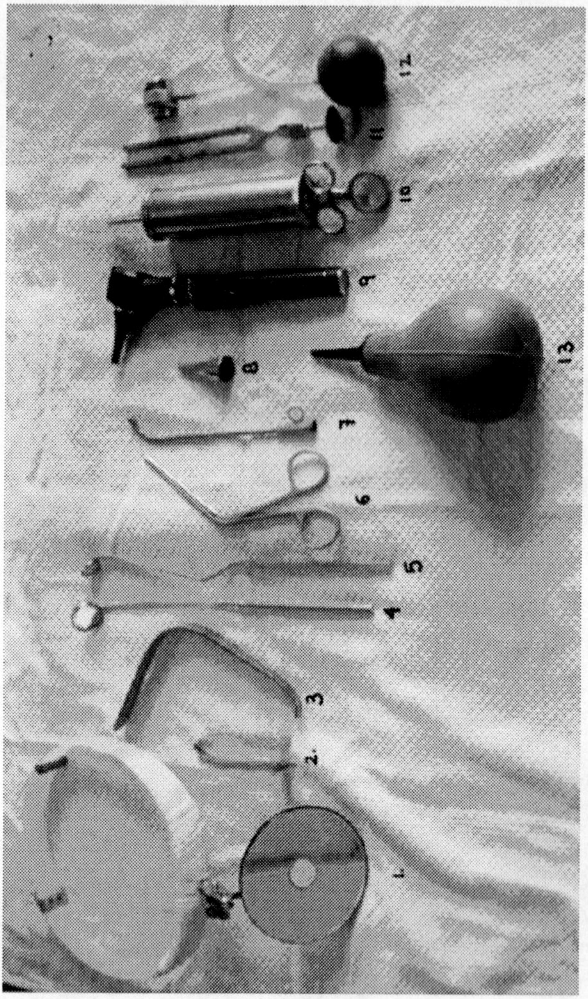

Fig 1: INSTRUMENTS USED IN OPD
Head mirror
Thudicum nasal speculum
Lack's tongue depressor
Indirect laryngoscopic mirror
Posterior rhinoscopy mirror
Nasal packing forceps
Eustachian catheter (Metallic)
Aural speculum
Otoscope
Aural syringe
Tuning fork
Siegle 's pneumatic speculum
Politzer bag

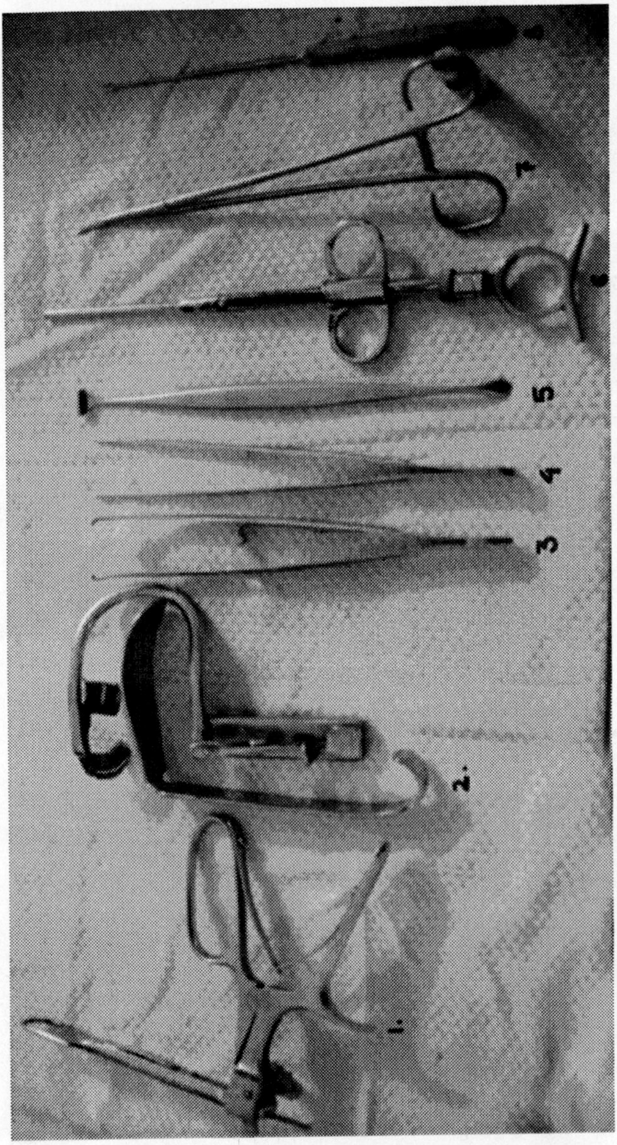

Fig 2: TONSILLECTOMY SET
1. Guillotine
2. Boyle Davis mouth gag with tongue piece
3. Tonsil holding forceps (Denis Browne)
4. Waugh's long dissecting forceps
5. Anterior pillar retractor with dissector
6. Eve's Tonsil snare with wire
7. Tonsillar artery forceps
8. Ligature slipper or knot tier

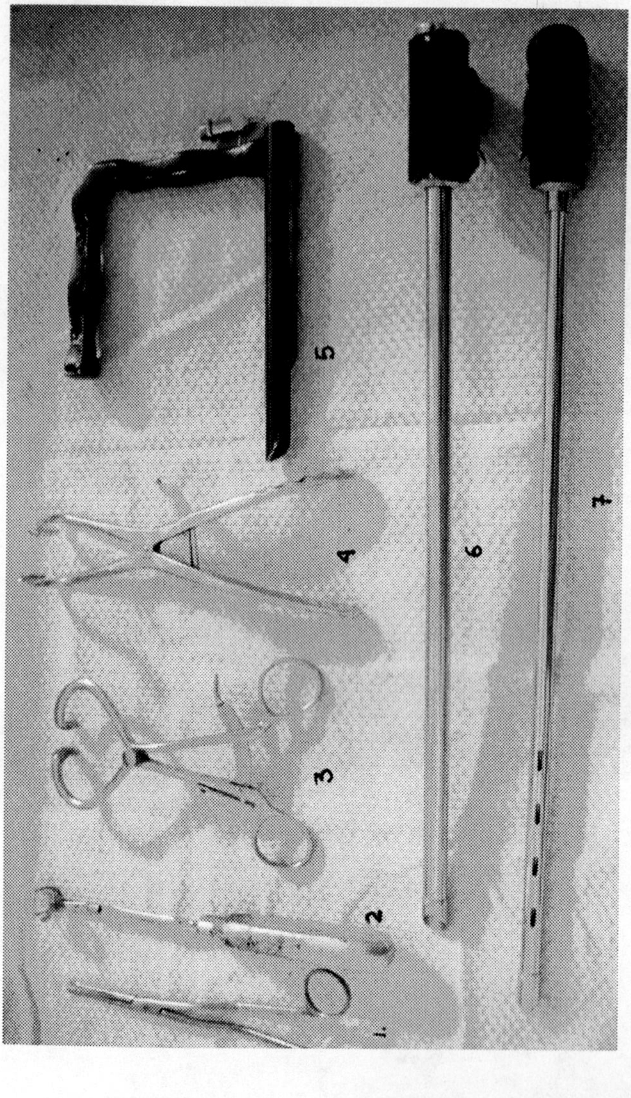

Fig 3: INSTRUMENTS FOR OTHER OPERATIONS IN THROAT:
Quinse or peritonsillar abscess forceps
St. Clair Thomson adenoid curette with cage
Doyne's mouth gag
Fergeuson's mouth gag
Direct laryngoscope
Oesophagoscope
Bronchoscope

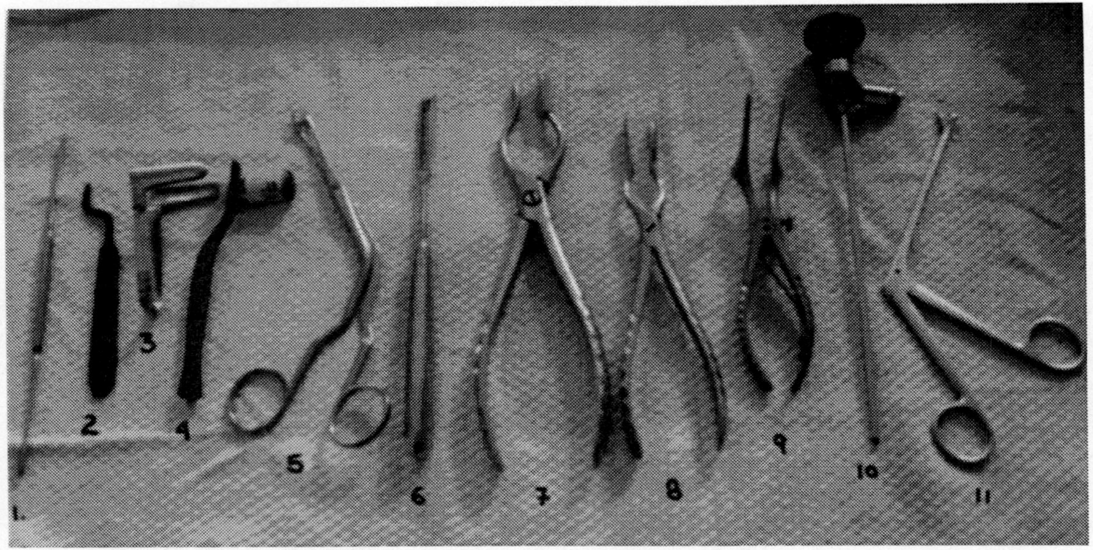

Fig 4: INSTRUMENTS USED IN VARIOUS NASAL OPERATIONS
Free muco-perichondrial elevator
Killian's muco-perichondrial elevator
Long bladed nasal speculum
Killian's Bayonet-shaped nasal gouge
Luc forceps
Ballenger's swivel knife
Walsham forceps
Asche's forceps
Duckbill nasal speculum
Nasal sinuscope
Blacklesley nasal forceps

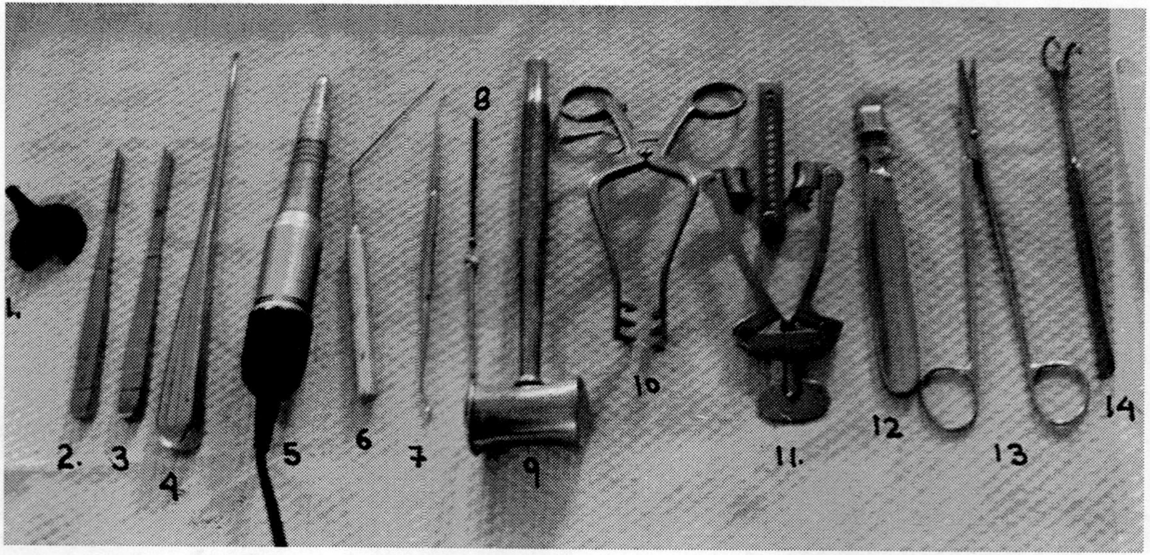

Fig 5: INSTRUMENT USED IN VARIOUS OPERATION OF THE EAR

Beveled aural speculum
Bone gouge
Chisel
Lempert's curette
Electric drill
Myringotomy knife
Aditus seeker with curette
Burr points / Drill bits
Mallet
Mollison's self retaining, haemostatic post aural retractor
Endaural Retractor
Periosteal elevator
Curved scissors
Double hook retractor

7

Radiology

(I) RADIOLOGY OF PARANASAL SINUS {Images 7-I-1 & 7-I-2}

Following are the 2 groups of paranasal sinuses that need to be evaluated radiologically

1. Anterior group of sinuses :
   (a) Maxillary
   (b) Anterior (& Middle) ethmoids
   (c) Frontal
2. Posterior group of sinuses :
   (a) Posterior ethmoids.
   (b) Sphenoids.

Following are the views that are needed to be known for the ENT practical examination :

1. X-ray PNS occiptomental view.
2. X-ray PNS occipitofrontal view.
3. X-ray skull lateral view.
4. X-ray skull submentovertical view.

Q. Why is this an occipitomental (OM) view?

A. Since the shadow of petrous apex overlaps the maxillary antrum this is a OF view. The position of plate in this view is touching the tip of the nose and the forehead simultaneously while the rays are incident from occipital end.

Q. Which sinuses are visualized in this OF view?

A. Mainly the frontal and ethmoid sinuses are visualized in OF view.

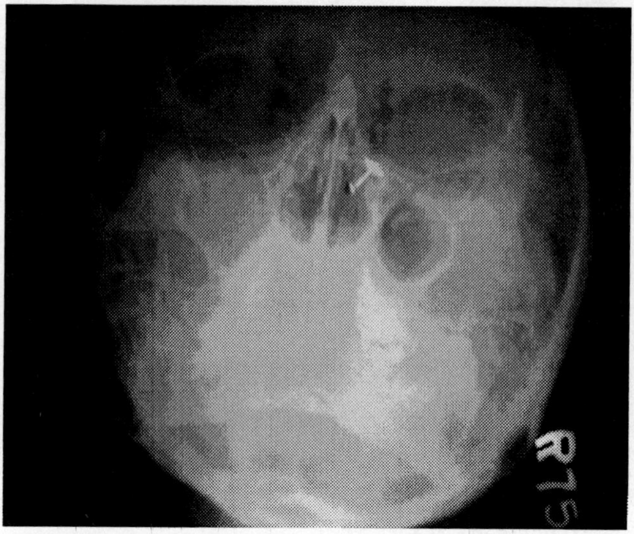

Fig. 7-I-1: Plain X-ray skull occipitomental view showing haziness of left maxillary sinus with normal contour suggestive of maxillary sinusitis (left).

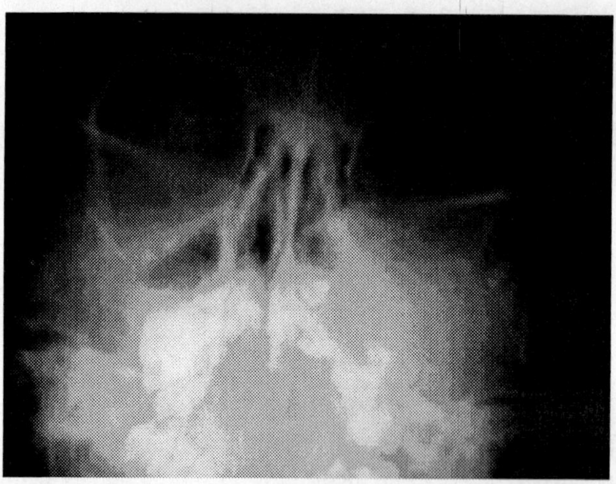

Fig. 7-I-2: Plain X-ray skull occipitomental view showing marked haziness of left maxillary sinus with bony erosion of anterolateral wall suggestive of malignancy maxilla (left). Note the enhancement and involvement of inferior orbital margin.

Since the proximity of frontal and ethmoid sinuses is more (close) to the plate, their visualization is better as compared to in the OM view.

Q. What are the sinuses that are seen on a lateral view of skull?

A. The frontal sinus, entire ethmoid gallery, maxillary sinuses and sphenoid sinuses are seen in this view. Here the sinuses that are seen, are overlapped with the corresponding sinuses of the other side.

Note

In OM view the shadow of petrous apex overlaps alveolar arch sparing the maxillary sinuses which can be clearly visualized. Here the X-ray plate is placed in approximation with the tip of nose and chin while the X-rays are incedent from occipital end. This view best visualized the maxillary sinuses. However if the radiography is done with open mouth, it may be possible to see the sphenoid sinuses.

Q. What are the sinuses that are seen on X-ray skull submento-vertical view?

A. Both the sphenoid sinuses, both the ethmoid galleries and both the maxillary sinuses are seen separately in this view.

Q. What is the position of the X-ray plate in submentovertical view?

A. The plate is positioned below the chin and the rays incident from the vertex (vertically down).

Q. What is the advantage of having 4 views for paranasal sinuses?

A. A single view gives a two-dimensional picture while a view perpendicular to the former gives a three-dimensional impression. For example, haziness of ethmoid sinus on one side on OM & OF view cannot define whether anterior or posterior cells are involved. It can only predict that there is haziness (or sinusitis) on right (or left side). The lateral view of skull would clarify if the entire ethmoid gallery is hazy or only the anterior (or posterior) group of sinuses are involved. Thus, exact location of the pathology can be defined.

On the other hand if there is bilateral ethmoid haziness on one of the PA views the simultaneous information obtained from X-ray skull lateral view would not clear the picture since the ethmoid galleries of both the sides are superimposed. In other words the haziness of ethmoid gallery appreciated on a lateral view skull would not define whether the pathology is right (or left) sided. Here lies the importance of submentovertical view where both the ethmoid galleries are visualized simultaneously therefore the role of different views of PNS is complementary to each other in terms of defining the pathology. Submentovertical view is not carried out routinely due to technical problems but is done wherever required.

Note

Usually in examinations OM & OF views are most frequently shown and one needs to properly read the radiograph. An example of OM view is as follows: This is a plain X-ray plate of paranasal sinus posteroanterior occiptiomental view showing the anterior group of sinuses viz. maxillary, frontal and ethmoid, the nasal cavity, the nasal turbinates, nasal septum, the orbit, alveolus and teeth. There is nasal septal deviation on the left side with haziness of left maxillary sinus. No other pathology can be appreciated. Hence my impression is that the patient is having deviated nasal septum on left side as associated with maxillary sinusitis on the left side as well.

To quickly read the X-ray one needs to see as many X-rays as possible along with the knowledge of the diagnostic features of probable pathologies (Table 7-I-1).

Table 7-I-1 :

X-ray findings	Diagnosis
1. Haziness of sinuses only	Sinusitis
2. Bony expansion without erosion	Benign tumefaction e.g. polyposis.
3. Decreased air shadow in nasal cavity without bony expansion	Hypertrophic rhinitis
4. Bony erosion with expansion	Malignancy
5. Bony defect without expansion or haziness	Surgically induced (iatrogenic) or fracture
6. Fluid level in maxillary sinus	Sinusitis with pus signifying acute bacterial maxillary sinusitis.

II. RADIOGRAPHIC DIAGNOSIS OF FRACTURE NASAL BONE

The following X-ray is ordered to document the fracture nasal bone: 'X-ray soft tissue of face, lateral view for fracture nasal bone.'

Q. What is this ? Comment upon.

A. This is a plan X-ray plate of the soft tissue of face, lateral view showing discontinuity in the nasal bone signifying a fracture.

Note

It should be noted whether the fractured segments are multiple or not. Accordingly, in the former case it would be better to call it a comminuted fracture. If there is a doubt or the quality of X-ray is very poor then there is no need to comment upon whether it is simple or comminuted (only use the word fracture).

Q. How many types (or classes) of fractures you know of?

A. Clinically there are three types of fractures. Class I fracture is the most simple and uncomplicated fracture due to a lateral blow on the nasal bone. The deformity is minimal and corrected easily. Class II fracture is more severe and occurs due to frontolateral below. Here there is a gross nasal deformity that needs surgical correction. Complications due to surrounding structure damage may be seen. Class III fracture is of the most severe variety often giving rise to complication due to surrounding structure damage and very significant external deformity. This is due to a frontal blow where the crushed nasal bone is pushed inside the ethmoidal air cells, and the patient presents with telecanthus (and gross facial deformity).

Note

Further details of clinical diagnosis and management can be asked and a standard textbook is to be consulted.

III. RADIOGRAPHIC DIAGNOSIS OF ENLARGED STYLOID PROCESS

The following X-ray is ordered to document an enlarged styloid process : "X-ray skull postero-anterior view with open month for enlarged styloid process'. It may be possible to have an X-ray showing enlarged styloid with closed mouth as well.

Q. What is this X-ray?

A. This is a plain X-ray plate of skull postero-anterior view with open mouth (watch for close mouth) showing enlarged styloid process. Probably the patient is suffering from stylalgia.

Q. How does the styloid process get enlarged?

A. The enlarged styloid process is the ossified part of stylohyoid ligament that is seen on X-ray.

Q. How does this ossification in the ligament lead to pain (stylalgia)?

A. The ossified ligament in continuity with the styloid process presents as a rigid structure irritating the surrounding pain sensitive structures such as glossopharyngeal nerve resulting into glossopharyngeal neuralgia.

Q. Is it possible that a rigid stylohyoid ligament can cause stylalgia?

A. The visualization on X-ray plate depends upon the degree of ossification. If the degree of ossification is not enough to reveal it on X-ray, it may still be rigid enough to cause irritation and thereby stylalgia.

Q. Is it possible to find an enlarged styloid process accidentally in an asymptomatic patient?

A. Theoretically yes but is quite unlikely.

Note

Further details of clinical diagnosis, management of stylalgia or enlarged styloid process can be asked and the student should consult a standard textbook accordingly.

IV. RADIOGRAPHIC DIAGNOSIS OF ENLARGED NASOPHARYNGEAL TONSILS (ADENOIDS)

The following X-ray is ordered to document adenoids : X-ray skull Lateral view of nasopharynx for adenoids'.

Q. What is this view and what is this showing?

A. This is a plain X-ray plate of skull lateral view showing nasopharynx with enlarged adenoids, filling up the nasopharynx and encroaching the upper end of choana (see the extent) and reducing the post-nasal space. The surrounding structures especially the nasal cavity, choana, skull base, sphenoid sinus and oropharynx are normal.

Note

The student is advised to consult a standard ENT textbook for clinical features (including adenoid facies) and management of adenoids that are likely to be asked also.

Q. What is the correlation between the size of adenoids and patient symptomatology?

A. Previously it was thought that larger the adenoids seen on plain X-ray, worse is the symptomatology and stronger are the indications for adenoidectomy. Recently several studies have specifically shown that size of adenoids on plain X-ray have poor correlation with the symptomatology. Hence the size of adenoids should be correlated with clinical sign and symptoms for planning surgery.

Note

Any bony erosion of skull base should suggest malignancy and NOT adenoids.

V. RADIOGRAPHIC DIAGNOSIS OF FOREIGN BODY IN DIGESTIVE TRACT {Images 7-V-1 & 7-V-2}

The foreign bodies in the digestive tract (pharyngeal and esophageal) are problematic only if impacted. In practical examinations, X-ray plate documenting a foreign body (mainly a coin) in lower end of

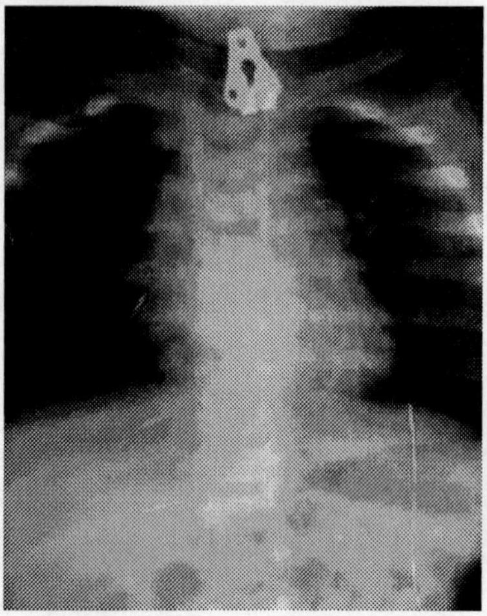

Fig. 7-V-1: Plain X-ray neck, chest and abdomen PA view showing a radio-opaque metallic (buckle) foreign body in esophagus. Note the tracheal air shadow besides the foreign body.

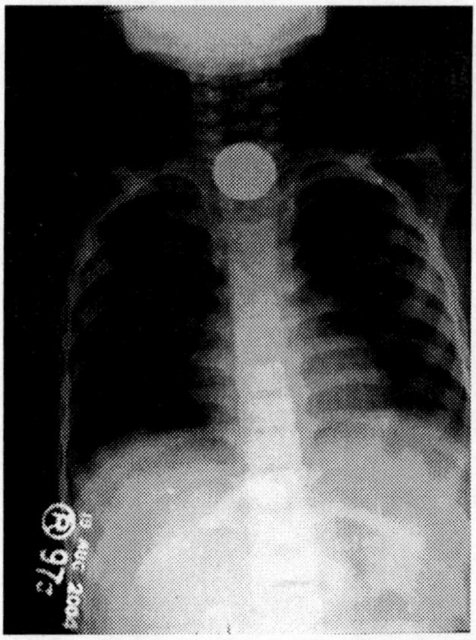

Fig. 7-V-2: Plain X-ray neck, thorax and upper abdomen (PA view) showing a round radio-opaque foreign body (metallic coin) impacted in the esophagus at the level of T-2/T-2.

pharynx or in esophagus is mostly asked. Theoretically the foreign body can be.

1. Animate – radioleucent
2. Inanimate
   (a) Vegetative – radioleucent
   (b) Non-vegetative, usually radio-opaque.

The radio-opaque foreign bodies are seen on plain X-ray PA view of neck or thorax but for documenting a radioleucent foreign body, a barium swallow examination would be needed to demonstrate a filling defect. After confirming the presence of foreign body, its extraction under general anesthesia by oesophagoscopy is planned as soon as possible.

Q. What is this x-ray showing?

A. This is a plain X-ray of neck including thorax PA view showing (type of) F.B. in digestive tract at the level of C5, 6, (or T 4,5 as per the findings).

Q. Why do you say that the coin is impacted in esophagus?

A. Firstly, a coin is too big to be impacted so lower down in primary bronchus. Secondly, the impaction of F.B. is in midline corresponding to the esophagus. Thirdly, the coin is lying in the coronal plane corresponding to the maximum transverse diameter of esophagus.

Q. What is the usual site of impaction for a F. B. in digestive tract?

A. The criopharynx is the narrowest part where impaction usually occurs. Once the F.B. has bypassed this obstacle, it is likely to pass out in stools. Still if F.B. does not show any signs of descent for another 24 hrs it is best extracted.

Q. How does the impaction of vegetative (or animate meat piece) foreign body differ from that of coin?

A. Any foreign body impacted in the esophagus gives rise to foreign body reaction resulting in inflammation at the site of impaction, ultimately leading to oesophagitis, perioesophagitis and esophageal perforation. Such reactions are manifold more severe in cases of organic foreign bodies due to release of chemicals. Hence it is essential to extract a vegetative / animate foreign body as soon as possible.

Note

1. Students are advised to consult standard ENT textbook for clinical features, management of an esophageal F. B. which can very well be asked along with X-ray.
2. A denture impaction in the esophagus is seen quite often. Careful examination of the plain X-ray would reveal a shadow of a wire along the length of esophagus.
3. Small object such as pin, safety pin, ear tops are sometimes seen in clinical practice. Only a careful examination in search of the above would clinch the diagnosis. Such small objects are as likely to be seen in esophagus as in the airway tract. Hence a careful assessment of the site of impaction is to be made before concluding the diagnosis.

VI. RADIOGRAPHIC DIAGNOSIS OF FOREIGN BODY (FB) IN AIRWAY TRACT {IMAGE 7-VI-1}

Foreign body impaction in airway tract is usually seen in children.

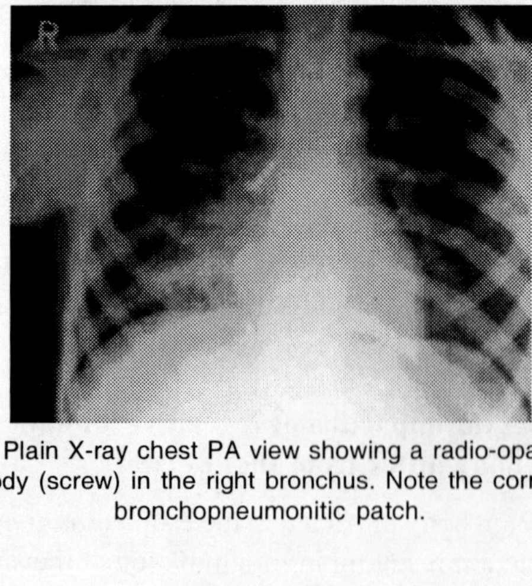

Fig. 7-VI-1: Plain X-ray chest PA view showing a radio-opaque metallic foreign body (screw) in the right bronchus. Note the corresponding bronchopneumonitic patch.

The foreign bodies usually seen in clinical practice are groundnuts, whistle, and other smaller metallic / plastic materials. The clinical features vary from relatively asymptomatic stage to the most severe form of respiratory distress (students are advised to consult a standard textbook). Any history of inhaled foreign body or even being suspicious of a F.B. inhalation (in an infant) in an otherwise asymptomatic patient should be urgently admitted and managed accordingly. Such cases should urgently undergo a bronchoscopy under general anesthesia for extraction of F.B. The relevance of chest X-ray is to see the presence of radio-opaque F. B. or to appreciate the pulmonary changes due to F.B. dynamics. The role of tracheostomy is to reduce the dead space, facilitate oxygenation and clear the excessive secretions for facilitating ventilation. For a glottic F. B. a tracheostomy bypassing the obstruction can be life saving.

Q. What is this X-ray showing?

A. This is a plain X-ray of neck and thorax PA view showing a small radio-opaque foreign body (see for the F.B.) in trachea.

Q. Why is the impaction of F.B. more in right bronchus as compared to left?

A. Since the right bronchus is more co-linear with the axis of trachea and is also somewhat wider the F.B. has a natural tendency of impacting in right bronchus.

Q. What can be the changes in lung parenchyma due to presence of F.B. in primary bronchus?

A. The foreign body in the primary bronchus can produce a total or a partial obstruction. A total obstruction would result into collapse of that particular lung gradually as the air would get observed with time. Hence a mediastinal shift to the same side would result. On the other hand partial obstruction of primary bronchus results in air trapping inside the lung as it allows air to enter inside the lung but prevent its exit during expiration. Such a ball-valve mechanism results in emphysema with mediastinal shift to the opposite side.

Q. What is the significance of mediastinal shift?

A. If the foreign body is radioleucent, a mediastinal shift is the only objective finding on X-ray suggestive of a F.B. in bronchus. Mediastinal shift to one side denotes either total collapse of the ipsilateral lung due to total obstruction of primary bronchus or an emphysema of the contralateral lung due to partial (ball valve) obstruction of primary bronchus.

Q. How will you extract the F.B.?

A. A bronchoscopy under general anesthesia is done in every suspicious case to locate and subsequently extract the F.B. by forceps.

VII. RADIOGRAPHIC ASSESSMENT OF TEMPORAL BONE PATHOLOGY IN MIDDLE EAR DISEASE {Images 7-VII-1 & 7-VII-2}

The following 2 radiographs for depicting temporal bone pathology in middle ear disease are most commonly asked in examinations.

1. X-ray skull AP- Towne's view for mastoid.
2. X-ray temporal bone Stenver's view.

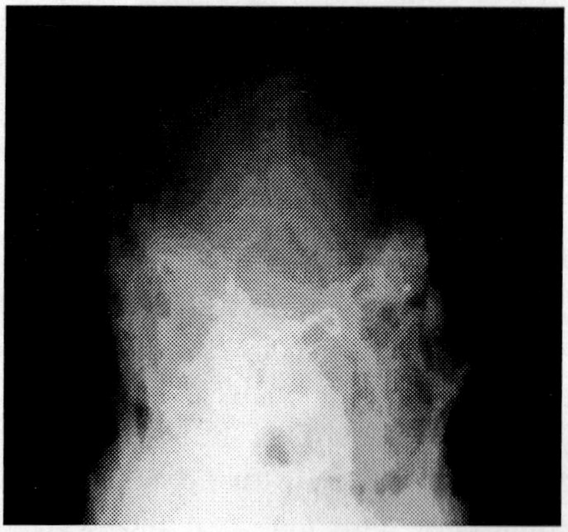

Fig. 7-VII-1: plain X-ray skull Towne's view for mastoid showing sclerotic mastoid on left side while on the right side an irregular large radioleucent shadow is present suggestive of previous surgery. (Note that the margins do NOT show any sclerosis or enhancement).

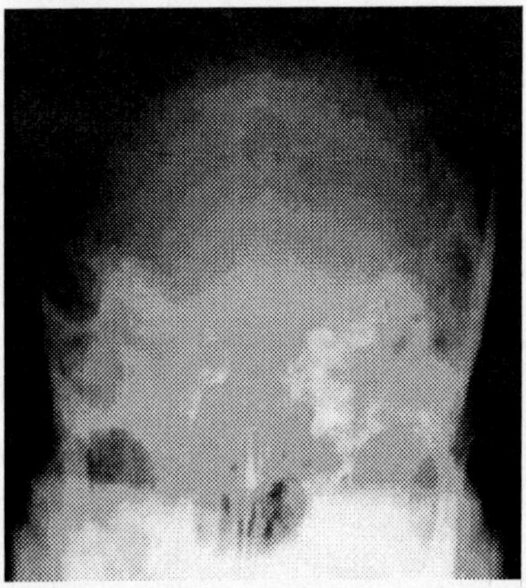

Fig. 7-VII-2: Plain X-ray skull Towne's view for mastoid showing a radioleucent oval shadow with radio-opaque enhanced (sclerosed) margins on right side suggestive of cholesteatoma. The mastoid on the left side has normal cellularity.

Following structures (landmarks) need to be carefully observed for : (1) Mastoid process (2) Mastoid air cells (3) External auditory canal (4) Middle ear space (5) ossicular shadow (6) Tegmen plate (7) Semicircular canals (8) Cochlea & (9) Internal auditory meatus.

Following pathology needs to be commented upon.

1. Mastoid air cell system may be either cellular (well defined air cells and septae), sclerotic (poorly defined air cells, sclerosis of mastoid) or mixed (combination of above two).
2. Cholesteatoma is radiographically characterized by radioleucent oral shadow with peripheral enhancement (sclerosis). Bony destruction may be present and air cell system is usually hazy.
3. Coalescent mastoiditis is seen radiographically as a radioleucent oval shadow without peripheral enhancement. The mastoid air cells coalesce to form a cavity following destruction of intercellular septae.
4. Malignancy, of temporal bone is characterized by an irregular soft tissue shadow with extensive bony destruction and loss of normal landmarks.
5. Iatrogenic surgical bony destruction is characterized by irregular (NOT OVAL) radioleucent shadow without peripheral enhancement and well-preserved residual normal landmarks.

8

Tuning Forks and Sample Audiograms

TUNING FORK

There are 3 parts of a tuning fork : Prongs, stem & base. The vibrations of prongs and base / stem are perpendicular to each other. Three types of tuning forks are used in clinical practice viz that of frequencies 256. Hz, 512 Hz & 1024 Hz. to characterize the hearing impairment. These are Weber test, Rinne test and Absolute bone conduction (ABC) test. For the methodology of elicitation of these tests, the reader is referred to a standard ENT text book.

Q. Which single (frequency) tuning fork would you select for screening of hearing impairment and why ?

A. For quick screening, the tuning fork with frequency 512 Hz would be most suitable because it represents the mid frequency range and its vibrations are sufficiently intense as well as prolonged to conclude the result. In contrast a 256 Hz tuning fork would produce a low pitched vibration like sound and that too for a shorter interval. On the other hand the sound produced by 1024 Hz tuning fork would although be long lasting but the intensity would be less.

Q. How will you say that the patient has conductive or sensory neural hearing impairment.

A. Decreased ABC signifies sensorineural deafness whatsoever. A negative Rinne's test is suggestive of conductive hearing loss. A combination of above suggests mixed deafness. (Students should have a thorough knowledge about interpretation of the tuning fork test and is referred to a standard textbook for the same.

Q. Which of the tuning fork tests is the most sensitive for detection of hearing loss.

A. Weber test is the most sensitive of all in detecting deafness to the tune of 5 dB. On the other hand Rinne's test can detect deafness to the tune of 10-15 dB.

Q. Based on tuning fork test how will you measure the degree (mild, moderate, severe) of conductive hearing loss ?

A. If Rinne's test with 256 Hz tuning fork is negative but that with 512 & 1024 Hz is positive the subject is said to have mild hearing loss. A moderate deafness on the other hand would be characterized by negative Rinne with 250 Hz and 512 Hz tuning forks but a positive Rinne's with 1024 Hz. Lastly, a severe conductive deafness would result in negative Rinne with all the tuning forks.

Note

For vibrating the tuning fork, the prongs should be struck on a firm surface such as the rigid hypothenar eminence of palm. Striking it on hard surface such as metal should be avoided as it would produce overtones.

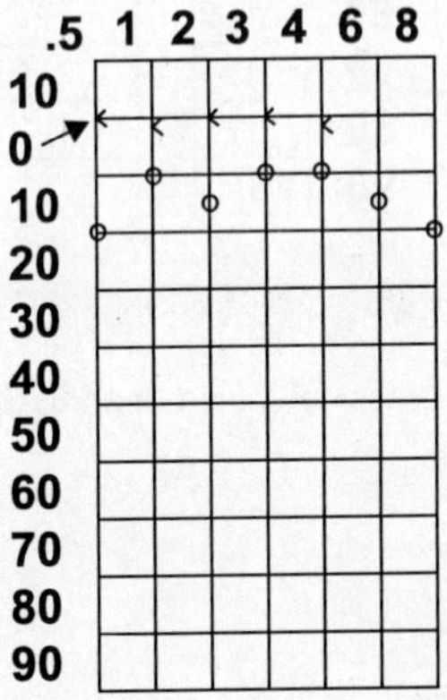

Fig 8-1: Normal hearing (Right)

Frequency (hertz) is charted horizontally from 0.5 to 8.0 kHz. While intensity in decibels is charted vertically from –5 to 100 dB and onwards. Threshold of hearing (minimum audible tone) is charted against each frequency and is subsequently joined, to give rise to the respective audiometric curve of the ear. The symbols representing the AC and BC of right and left ears are as follows:

O : AC for right ear
X : AC for left ear
< : BC for right ear
> : BC for left ear

The Figure 8-1 shows.

Air conduction (AC) threshold (average of AC at 0.5, 1, 2, & 4 kHz.) = < 15

Bone conduction threshold (BC) < 5

AB gap (AC threshold – BC threshold) = 10

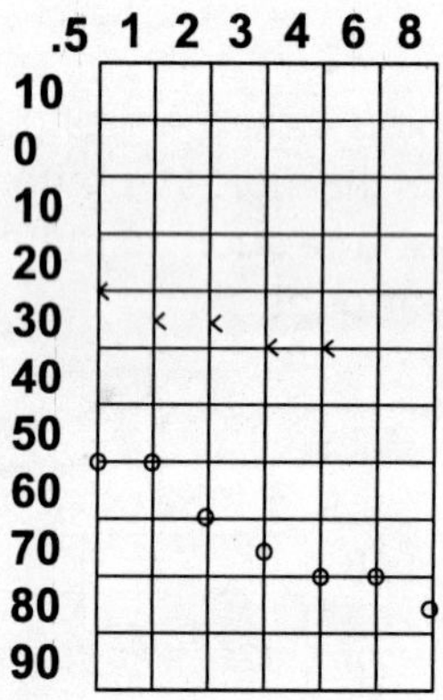

AC = 65 BC = 35 AB gap = 30

Fig. 8-2: Classical mixed hearing loss (Right ear)

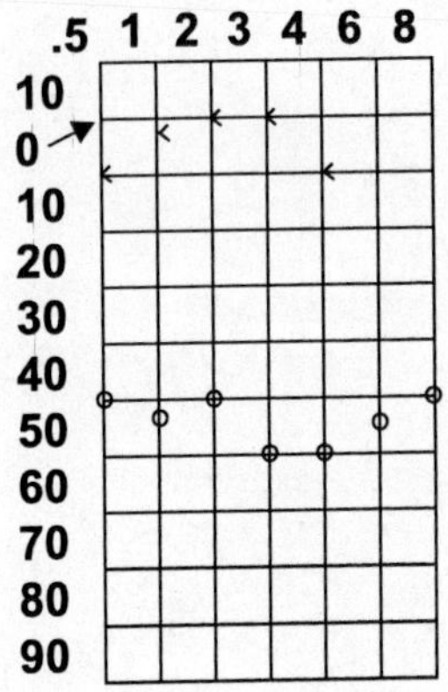

AC > 50 BC < 10 AB gap > 40

Fig. 8-3. Classical conductive hearing loss (Right ear)

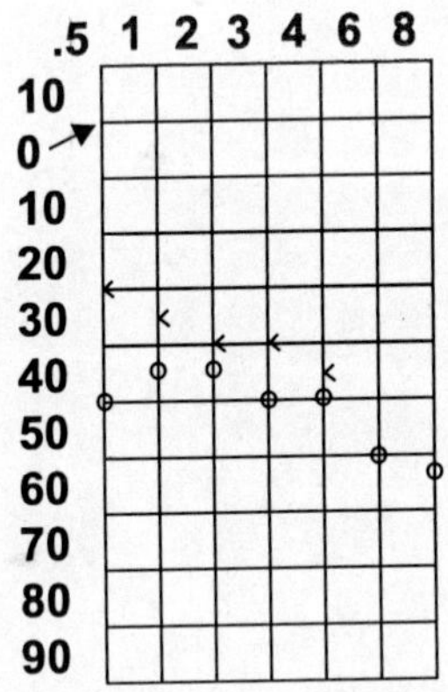

BC > 35 AB gap < 10

Fig 8-4: Classical sensorineural hearing loss (Right ear).